Donald S. Fong

Simon K. Law

Ursula Schmidt-Erfurth

Editors

Drugs in Ophthalmology

T0186026

Donald S. Fong
Simon K. Law
Ursula Schmidt-Erfurth

Editors

Drugs in Ophthalmology

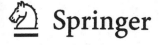 Springer

Donald S. Fong, MD, MPH
Director
Clinical Trials
Department of Research and Evaluation
Kaiser Permanente Southern California
100 S. Los Robles
Pasadena
CA 91101, USA

Ursula Schmidt-Erfurth, MD
Professor and Chair
Department of Ophthalmology
Medical University of Vienna
Währinger Gürtel 18–20
A-1090 Vienna, Austria

Simon K. Law, MD, PharmD
Jules Stein Eye Institute
100 Stein Plaza 2-235
Los Angeles
CA 90095, USA

ISBN-10 3-540-23435-7 Springer-Verlag Berlin Heidelberg New York
ISBN-13 978-3-540-23435-7 Springer-Verlag Berlin Heidelberg New York

Library of Congress Control Number: 2005933261

Springer is a part of Springer Science+Business Media
springeronline.com
© Springer-Verlag Berlin Heidelberg 2006
Printed in Germany

Editor: Marion Philipp, Heidelberg, Germany
Desk Editor: Martina Himberger, Heidelberg, Germany
Production: ProEdit GmbH, Heidelberg, Germany
Cover: Frido Steinen-Broo, EStudio Calamar, Spain
Typesetting: Stürtz GmbH, Würzburg, Germany

Printed on acid-free paper 24/3151 Re 5 4 3 2 1 0

Disclaimer

The nature of drug information is that it is constantly changing because of continuing research and clinical experience and is often subject to ongoing evaluation. While significant care has been taken to ensure the accuracy of the information, the reader is advised that the authors, editors, reviewers, contributors, and publishers cannot be responsible for the continued currency of the information, for any errors or omissions in this book, or for any consequences arising therefrom. Because of the changing nature of drug information, readers are advised that decisions regarding drug therapy must be based on the independent judgment of the ophthalmologist, changing information (literature and manufacturer's information), and changing medical practice.

List of Contributors

Amani A. Fawzi, MD
  University of Southern California
  Keck School of Medicine
  Doheny Eye Institute
  San Pablo Street 1450
  Los Angeles
  CA 90033, USA

Donald S. Fong, MD, MPH
  Director
  Clinical Trials
  Department of Research and Evaluation
  Kaiser Permanente Southern California
  100 S. Los Robles
  Pasadena
  CA 91101, USA

Simon K. Law, MD, PharmD
  Jules Stein Eye Institute
  100 Stein Plaza 2-235
  Los Angeles
  CA 90095, USA

Rike Michels
  Department of Ophthalmology
  Medical University of Vienna
  Währinger Gürtel 18–20
  A-1090 Vienna, Austria

Ursula Schmidt-Erfurth, MD
  Professor and Chair
  Department of Ophthalmology
  Medical University of Vienna
  Währinger Gürtel 18–20
  A-1090 Vienna, Austria

Hasan Syed, MD, Stanford University
  Medical Center
  General Surgery
  Welch Road 1170
  Palo Alto
  CA 94304, USA

Table of Contents

Introduction

This drug handbook is divided into two sections:

Alphabetical Listing of Drugs
Entries in this section are listed by generic name. Information for each drug is arranged in a consistent format for easy reference. If one or more of the following categories is not applicable to a certain drug, it will not be listed. If *Pregnancy Category* is not listed for an individual drug, then it is either listed under the first drug in a group of drugs, or safety and efficacy in pregnancy have not been established.

Summary of Anti-infectives
This section summarizes the common doses of antibiotics, antifungals, and antivirals. For each drug, the dose for each route of administration is included.

Generic name	
Brand names	Common trade names
Class of drug	Therapeutic class
Indications	Common uses of the drug
Dosage form	Common forms of the drug
Dose	The amount of drug to be given or taken during therapy. The dosage is to be taken as a guideline and does not preclude other dosage regimens
Contraindications	Information pertaining to inappropriate use of the drug
Warnings	Hazardous conditions related to use of the drug and disease states or patient populations in which the drug should be used cautiously
Adverse reactions	Considerations to be taken into account
Pregnancy category	FDA categories that indicate the potential for causing birth defects
A	Controlled studies in pregnant women have failed to demonstrate a risk to the fetus in the first trimester with no evidence of risk in later trimesters. The possibility of fetal harm appears remote
B	Either animal-reproduction studies have not demonstrated a fetal risk but there are no controlled studies in pregnant women, or animal-reproduction studies have shown an adverse effect that was not confirmed in controlled studies in women in the first trimester and there was no evidence of a risk in later trimesters
C	Either studies in animals have revealed adverse effects on the fetus (teratogenic, embryocidal effects, or other) and there are no controlled studies in women, or studies in women and animals are not available. Drugs should be given only if the potential benefits justify the potential risk to the fetus
D	There is positive evidence of human fetal risk, but the benefits from use in pregnant women may be acceptable despite the risk (e.g., if the drug is needed in a life-threatening situation or for a serious disease for which safer drugs cannot be used or are ineffective)

Generic name	
X	Studies in animals or humans have demonstrated fetal abnormalities or there is evidence of fetal risk based on human experience, or both, and the risk of the use of the drug in pregnant women clearly outweighs any possible benefit. The drug is contraindicated in women who are or may become pregnant
Drug interactions	Only clinically important interactions are listed

Alphabetical Listing of Drugs

Acetazolamide

Brand Name	Diamox.
Class of Drug	Carbonic anhydrase inhibitor (CAI) (sulfonamide).
Indications	Benign intracranial hypertension, ocular hypertension, open-angle glaucoma (OAG), secondary glaucoma, preoperatively in acute angle-closure glaucoma (ACG), some forms of cystoid macular edema, acute mountain sickness.
Dosage Form	*Oral*: 125 mg, 250 mg. *IV*: 500 mg/vial.
Dose	*Glaucoma*: should be used as adjunct to usual therapy; 250 mg to 1 g/24 h in adults. *Secondary glaucoma, or preoperatively in acute ACG to delay surgery*: 250 mg every 4 h (some reported cases of short-term efficacy with 250 mg b.i.d.). *Acute cases*: Initial 500 mg dose followed by 125–250 mg every 4 h. In benign intracranial hypertension, initial dose should not be less than 1 g/day. IV therapy may be used for rapid relief of ocular hypertension.
Contraindications	In patients with decreased serum sodium and/or potassium, marked renal or hepatic disease/dysfunction, suprarenal gland failure, hyperchloremic acidosis, liver cirrhosis, or for long-term use for ACG.
Warnings	Discontinue use if hypersensitivity develops. Rare fatalities have occurred due to severe sulfonamide reactions (Stevens–Johnson syndrome, toxic epidermal necrolysis, fulminant hepatic necrosis, agranulocytosis, aplastic anemias, and other blood dyscrasias). In patients with pulmonary obstruction or emphysema where alveolar ventilation may be impaired, it may aggravate acidosis and should be used with caution.
Adverse Reactions	*May occur*: (common to all sulfonamide derivatives): anaphylaxis, fever, rash (including erythema multiforme, Stevens-Johnson syndrome, toxic epidermal necrolysis), crystalluria, renal calculus, bone-marrow depression, thrombocytopenic purpura, hemolytic anemia, leukopenia, pancytopenia, agranulocytosis, (precaution is advised for early detection of such reactions, and the drug should be discontinued and appropriate therapy instituted), paresthesias, tinnitus, decreased appetite, taste alteration, gastrointestinal (GI) symptoms (nausea, vomiting, diarrhea), polyuria, drowsiness, confusion, metabolic acidosis, electrolyte imbalance, increased or decreased blood glucose levels, transient myopia (subsides after discontinuation), *Occasional*: urticaria, melena, hematuria, glycosuria, hepatic insufficiency, flaccid paralysis, photosensitivity, convulsions.
	Periodic monitoring for hematologic reactions and electrolyte imbalance with a baseline complete blood count (CBC) and platelet count and serum electrolytes are recommended prior to initiating therapy and at regular intervals during therapy. If significant changes occur, early discontinuance and institution of appropriate therapy are important.
Pregnancy Category	C.

Drug Interactions	Safety and effectiveness in pediatric patients have not been established. Growth retardation has been reported in children receiving long-term therapy believed secondary to chronic acidosis. Caution advised for patients on concomitant high-dose aspirin (reported cases of anorexia, tachypnea, lethargy, coma, death). Modifies phenytoin metabolism with increased serum levels of phenytoin. May decrease serum concentrations of primidone and its metabolites by decreasing the absorption of primidone. May increase the effects of other folic acid antagonists. May reduce urinary excretion of amphetamine and quinidine and prevent the urinary antiseptic effect of methenamine. May increase lithium excretion. May elevate cyclosporine level.

Brand Name	Diamox Sequels.
Class of Drug	Sustained release.
Indications	See »Diamox.«
Dosage Form	Sustained-release capsules 500 mg.
Dose	Glaucoma: 500 mg capsule two times per day (A.M., P.M.).
Contraindications	See »Diamox.«
Warnings	See »Diamox.«
Adverse Reactions	See »Diamox.«
Pregnancy Category	C.
Drug Interactions	See »Diamox.«

Acetylcholine Chloride

Brand Name	Miochol-E.
Class of Drug	Miotic cholinergic.
Indications	Immediate miosis after lens placement in cataract surgery, penetrating keratoplasty, iridectomy, other anterior segment surgery where rapid miosis is desired.*Off-label*: acetylcholine has been used without approval in cases of acute retinal vascular occlusion as a retrobulbar injection to relieve vasodilation of the retinal and choroidal blood vessels.
Dosage Form	Ophthalmic injection.*Intraocular upper chamber*: 20 mg acetylcholine and 56 mg mannitol. *Lower chamber*: 2 ml modified diluent.
Dose	0.5–2 ml intraocularly.
Contraindications	None known.
Warnings	Do not gas sterilize. Aqueous solutions are unstable. Prepare solution immediately before use and discard any solution that has not been used. Do not use solution that is not clear and colorless.

Adverse Reactions	*Infrequent*: corneal edema/clouding/decompensations. *Rare*: bradycardia, hypotension, flushing, breathing difficulties, sweating (all indicative of systemic absorption).
Pregnancy Category	C.
Drug Interactions	A few reports of interference in efficacy with use of topical nonsteroidal anti-inflammatory drugs (NSAIDs).

Acetylcysteine

Brand Name	Mucomyst; Mucosil 10% and 20%.
Class of Drug	Collagenase inhibitor. Mucolytic agent.
Indications	Off-label: alkali burns, corneal melts, and keratoconjunctivitis sicca, filamentary keratopathy, zoster mucous plaque keratitis.
Dosage Form	Ophthalmic solution 10% or 20%. Off-label: dilute the commercial preparation to 2–5% by adding artificial tears or physiologic saline.
Dose	1–2 drops to affected eye(s) up to four times per day in maintenance therapy and up to hourly in acute cases. (Commercially available solution is not approved for ophthalmic use.)
Pregnancy Category	B.

Acyclovir Sodium

Brand Name	Zovirax.
Class of Drug	Antiviral.
Indications	*Injection*: initial and recurrent mucosal and cutaneous herpes simplex virus (HSV-1 and HSV-2) in immunocompromised patients, severe initial clinical episodes of herpes genitalis in immunocompetent patients, herpes simplex encephalitis, neonatal herpes infections, varicella-zoster (shingles) infections in immunocompromised patients. *Capsules, tablets, suspension*: acute treatment of herpes zoster (shingles), initial episodes and management of recurrent episodes of genital herpes, varicella (chickenpox). *Ointment 5%*: initial genital herpes, limited non-life-threatening mucocutaneous, HSV infections in immunocompromised patients.
Dosage Form	See »Antivirals.«

Dose

HSV-1 and HSV-2 infections in immunocompromised patients: Adults and adolescents (12 years of age and older)—5 mg/kg infused at a constant rate over 1 h every 8 h for 7 days. Pediatrics (younger than 12 years of age)—10 mg/kg infused at a constant rate over 1 h every 8 h for 7 days. *Severe initial clinical episodes of herpes genitalis*: Adults and adolescents (12 years of age and older)—5 mg/kg infused at a constant rate over 1 h every 8 h for 5 days. *Herpes simplex encephalitis*: Adults and adolescents (12 years of age and older)—10 mg/kg infused at a constant rate over 1 h every 8 h for 10 days. Pediatrics (3 months to 12 years of age)—20 mg/kg infused at a constant rate over 1 h every 8 h for 10 days. *Neonatal HSV infections (birth to 3 months)*: 10 mg/kg infused at a constant rate over 1 h every 8 h for 10 days. In neonatal herpes simplex infections, doses of 15 mg/kg or 20 mg/kg (infused at a constant rate over 1 h every 8 h) have been used; safety and efficacy of these doses are not known. *Varicella-zoster infections in immunocompromised patients*: Adults and adolescents (12 years of age and older)—10 mg/kg infused at a constant rate over 1 h every 8 h for 7 days. Pediatrics (younger than 12 years of age)—20 mg/kg infused at a constant rate over 1 h every 8 h for 7 days. *Obese patients*: dose at the recommended adult dose using ideal body weight; dosage adjustments required for patients with renal impairment or undergoing hemodialysis. *Peritoneal dialysis*: no supplemental dose appears to be necessary after adjustment of the dosing interval.

Contraindications

In patients who develop hypersensitivity to the product or any of its components. *Cream*: intended for cutaneous use only and should not be used in the eye or inside the mouth or nose; should only be used on herpes labialis on the affected external aspects of the lips and face. *Ointment*: no data to support the use of Zovirax ointment 5% to prevent transmission of infection to other persons or prevent recurrent infections when applied in the absence of signs and symptoms; should not be used for the prevention of recurrent HSV infections.

Warnings

Renal failure, in some cases resulting in death, has been observed. Thrombotic thrombocytopenic purpura/hemolytic uremic syndrome (TTP/HUS), which has resulted in death, has occurred in immunocompromised patients. Abnormal renal function [decreased creatinine clearance (CrCl)] can occur as a result of administration and depends on the state of the patient's hydration, other treatments, and the rate of drug administration. Concomitant use of other nephrotoxic drugs and in patients with preexisting renal disease and dehydration make further renal impairment more likely. IV infusions must be given over a period of at least 1 h to reduce the risk of renal tubular damage. Approximately 1% of patients receiving i.v. acyclovir have manifested encephalopathic changes characterized by either lethargy, obtundation, tremors, confusion, hallucinations, agitation, seizures, or coma. Should be used with caution in those patients who have underlying neurologic abnormalities and those with serious renal, hepatic, or electrolyte abnormalities, or significant hypoxia.

Adverse Reactions
Most frequent: inflammation or phlebitis at the injection site; transient elevations of serum creatinine or blood urea nitrogen (BUN); nausea and/or vomiting; itching, rash, or hives; elevation of transaminases. *Less frequent*: anemia, neutropenia, thrombocytopenia, thrombocytosis, leukocytosis, neutrophilia, anorexia, and hematuria. *Others reported during clinical practice*: General—anaphylaxis, angioedema, fever, headache, pain, peripheral edema, fatigue. Digestive—diarrhea, gastrointestinal distress, nausea, abdominal pain. Cardiovascular—hypotension. Hematologic and lymphatic—disseminated intravascular coagulation, hemolysis, leukocytoclastic vasculitis, leukopenia, lymphadenopathy. Hepatobiliary tract and pancreas—elevated liver function tests (LFTs), hepatitis, hyperbilirubinemia, jaundice. Musculoskeletal—myalgia. Nervous system—aggressive behavior, agitation, ataxia, coma, confusion, delirium, dizziness, encephalopathy, hallucinations, obtundation, paresthesia, psychosis, seizure, somnolence, tremor, dysarthria (these symptoms may be marked, particularly in older adults). Skin—alopecia, erythema multiforme, photosensitive rash, pruritus, rash, Stevens–Johnson syndrome, toxic epidermal necrolysis, urticaria (severe local inflammatory reactions, including tissue necrosis, have occurred following infusion into extravascular tissues). Special senses—visual abnormalities. Urogenital—renal failure, elevated blood urea nitrogen, elevated creatinine.

Pregnancy Category
Drug Interactions
See »Antivirals.«

Adalimumab

Brand Name
Humira.

Class of Drug
Immunomodulator. Adalimumab binds specifically to tumor necrosis factor (TNF)-alpha and blocks its interaction with p55 and p75 cell-surface TNF receptors.

Indications
Rheumatoid arthritis.

Dosage Form
Solution for s.c. injection 40 mg/0.8 ml.

Dose
SC injection 40 mg every 2 weeks.

Contraindications
In patients with a known hypersensitivity to the product or any of its components.

Warnings
Serious and potentially fatal infections and sepsis have occurred in the setting of TNF-alpha blockade, including tuberculosis, histoplasmosis, listeriosis, and pneumocystosis. Lym-

phomas have been observed in patients treated with TNF-blocking agents, including adalimumab. Use of TNF-blocking agents has been associated with rare cases of exacerbation of clinical symptoms and/or radiographic evidence of demyelinating disease.

Adverse Reactions *Most serious*: serious infections, neurologic events, malignancies. *Most common*: injection-site erythema and/or itching, hemorrhage, pain, or swelling.

Pregnancy Category B.

Drug Interactions Safety and effectiveness in pediatric patients have not been established.

Amikacin Sulfate

Brand Name Amikin.

Class of Drug Antibiotic.

Indications Bacterial meningitis, pneumonia, septicemia, urinary tract infection (UTI), biliary tract infections, bone infections, burn-wound infections. Gram-negative aerobic bacillary pneumonia, intra-abdominal infection, joint infections. Neonatal meningitis, pneumonia, septicemia. Nosocomial pneumonia. *Acinetobacter*-complicated UTI, *Enterobacter* spp.-complicated UTI, *Escherichia coli*-complicated UTI, *Klebsiella* spp.-complicated UTI, *Proteus* spp.-complicated UTI, *Pseudomonas aeruginosa*-complicated UTI, *Serratia* spp.-complicated UTI. *Acinetobacter* biliary tract infection, joint infection, meningitis, osteomyelitis, pneumonia. *Enterobacter* biliary tract infection, meningitis, peritonitis, pneumonia, septicemia; *Enterobacter spp.* joint infection, osteomyelitis, skin and soft tissue infection. *E. coli* joint infection, osteomyelitis, peritonitis, septicemia, skin and soft tissue infection, biliary tract infection, meningitis, pneumonia. *Klebsiella* biliary tract infection, osteomyelitis, pneumonia, septicemia, *K. pneumoniae* peritonitis; *Klebsiella* spp. joint infection, skin and soft tissue infection, meningitis. *Proteus* biliary tract infection, meningitis, osteomyelitis, septicemia; *Proteus* spp. joint infection, peritonitis, pneumonia, skin and soft tissue infection. *P. aeruginosa* biliary tract infection, joint infection, meningitis, osteomyelitis, peritonitis, pneumonia, septicemia. *Serratia* biliary tract infection, meningitis, peritonitis, pneumonia, septicemia; *Serratia* spp. joint infection, osteomyelitis, skin and soft tissue infection. *Staphylococcus aureus* meningitis, pneumonia, septicemia, joint infection, osteomyelitis, skin and soft tissue infection; *Staphylococcus* spp. peritonitis. Synergy for bacterial meningitis, neonatal meningitis, nosocomial pneumonia due to *P. aeruginosa*, staphylococcal endocarditis, staphylococcal infections.

Dosage Form

Dose *Adult minimum:maximum*: 15.0 mg/kg:30.0 mg/kg. *Pediatric minimum:maximum*: 15.0 mg/kg:30.0 mg/kg.

Contraindications *Drug combination*: clearly contraindicated in all the following cases and should not be dispensed or administered to the same patient—antibiotics/live vaccines; decreased effect of the latter drug. *Most significant toxicity*: pregnancy. *Others*: significant dehydration, disorder of the eighth cranial nerve, hypocalcemia, infant botulism, myasthenia gravis, Parkinsonism, renal disease, tinnitus, vertigo.

Warnings *Pediatric relative contraindication*: monitor for neuromuscular blockage, central nervous system (CNS) depression or toxicity. *Lactation*: no known risk; no documented problems in humans; aminoglycosides are poorly absorbed. *Pregnancy*: not recommended. *Geriatric precaution*: monitor renal function; hearing loss possible even if normal.

Adverse Reactions *Most frequent*: auditory neurotoxicity, CNS toxicity, nephrotoxicity, ototoxicity, renal disease. *Less frequent*: allergic dermatitis, allergic reactions, angioedema, erythema, pruritus, skin rash. *Rare*: neuromuscular blockade, drug interactions.

Pregnancy Category D.

Drug Interactions Should be used with caution in premature and neonatal infants because of the renal immaturity of these patients and the resulting prolongation of serum half-life of the drug.

Amphotericin B

Brand Name Am B isome for injection (liposomal amphotericin B).

Class of Drug Antifungal.

Indications Empirical therapy for presumed fungal infection in febrile, neutropenic patients; treatment of cryptococcal meningitis in HIV-infected patients. Treatment of patients with *Aspergillus* spp., *Candida* spp. and/or *Cryptococcus* spp. infections (see above for the treatment of cryptococcal meningitis) refractory to amphotericin B deoxycholate or in patients where renal impairment or unacceptable toxicity precludes the use of amphotericin B deoxycholate. Treatment of visceral leishmaniasis. In immunocompromised patients with visceral leishmaniasis treated with Am B isome, relapse rates are high following initial clearance of parasites.

Dosage Form Intravenous.

Dose *Recommended initial dose for each indication for adult and pediatric patients*: Empirical therapy—3.0 mg/kg per day.

Systemic fungal infections—3.0–5.0 mg/kg per day *(Aspergillus, Candida, Cryptococcus)*. Cryptococcal meningitis in HIV-infected patients—6.0 mg/kg per day. Immunocompetent patients (visceral leishmaniasis)—3.0 mg/kg per day on days 1–5, and 3.0 mg/kg per day on days 14 and 21. Immunocompromised patients (visceral leishmaniasis)—4.0 mg/kg per day on days 1–5, and 4.0 mg/kg per day on days 10, 17, 24, 31, and 38.

Contraindications
In patients who have demonstrated or have known hypersensitivity to the product or any of its components unless, in the opinion of the treating physician, the benefit of therapy outweighs the risk.

Warnings
Anaphylaxis has been reported with amphotericin B deoxycholate and other amphotericin B-containing drugs. If a severe anaphylactic reaction occurs, the infusion should be immediately discontinued and the patient should not receive further infusions. Immediate treatment of anaphylaxis or anaphylactoid reactions is required.

Adverse Reactions
Body as a whole: abdominal pain, asthenia, back pain, blood product transfusion reaction, chills, infection, pain, sepsis, *Cardiovascular system*: chest pain, hypertension, hypotension, tachycardia. *Digestive system*: diarrhea, gastrointestinal hemorrhage, nausea, vomiting. *Metabolic and nutritional disorders*: alkaline phosphatase increased, alanine aminotransferase (ALT) [serum glutamic-pyruvic transaminase (SGPT)] increased, aspartate aminotransferase (AST) [serum glutamic-oxaloacetic transaminase (SGOT)] increased, bilirubinemia, BUN increased, creatinine increased, edema, hyperglycemia, hypernatremia, hypervolemia, hypocalcemia, hypokalemia, hypomagnesemia, peripheral edema. *Nervous system*: anxiety, confusion, headache, insomnia. *Respiratory system*: cough increased, dyspnea, epistaxis, hypoxia, lung disorder, pleural effusion, rhinitis. *Skin and appendages*: pruritus, rash, sweating. *Urogenital system*: hematuria.

Pregnancy Category
B.

Drug Interactions
Antineoplastic agents: Concurrent use may enhance the potential for renal toxicity, bronchospasm, and hypotension; should be given concomitantly with caution. *Corticosteroids and corticotropin (ACTH)*: Concurrent use may potentiate hypokalemia, which could predispose the patient to cardiac dysfunction; if used concomitantly, serum electrolytes and cardiac function should be closely monitored. *Digitalis glycosides*: Concurrent use may induce hypokalemia and potentiate digitalis toxicity; when administered concomitantly, serum potassium levels should be closely monitored. *Flucytosine*: Concurrent use may increase toxicity of flucytosine by possibly increasing its cellular uptake and/or impairing its renal excretion. *Azoles (e.g., ketoconazole, miconazole, clotrimazole, fluconazole, etc.)*:In vitro and in vivo animal studies suggest that imidazoles may induce fungal resistance to amphoteri-

cin B; combination therapy should be administered with caution, especially in immunocompromised patients. *Leukocyte transfusions*: Acute pulmonary toxicity has been reported in patients receiving leukocyte transfusions. *Other nephrotoxic medications*: Concurrent use with other nephrotoxic medications may enhance the potential for drug-induced renal toxicity; intensive monitoring of renal function is recommended in patients requiring any combination of nephrotoxic medications. *Skeletal muscle relaxants*: Amphotericin B-induced hypokalemia may enhance the curariform effect of skeletal muscle relaxants (e.g., tubocurarine) due to hypokalemia; when administered concomitantly, serum potassium levels should be closely monitored

Brand Name	Abelcet injection (amphotericin B lipid complex).
Class of Drug	Antifungal.
Indications	Invasive fungal infections in patients who are refractory to or intolerant of conventional amphotericin B therapy.
Dosage Form	Intravenous.
Dose	Recommended daily dose for adults and children: 5 mg/kg given as a single infusion.
Contraindications	In patients who have shown hypersensitivity to the product or any of its components.
Warnings	See »Am B isome for injection.« *Precautions*: General—as with any amphotericin B-containing product, during the initial dosing, the drug should be administered under close clinical observation by medically trained personnel. Acute reactions, including fever and chills, may occur 1–2 h after starting an i.v. infusion. These reactions are usually more common with the first few doses and generally diminish with subsequent doses. Infusion has been rarely associated with hypotension, bronchospasm, arrhythmias, and shock. Laboratory tests—serum creatinine should be monitored frequently during therapy. It is also advisable to regularly monitor liver function, serum electrolytes (particularly magnesium and potassium), and CBCs.
Adverse Reactions	Chills, fever, increased serum creatinine, multiple organ failure, nausea, vomiting, hypotension, respiratory failure, dyspnea, sepsis, diarrhea, headache, heart arrest, hypertension, hypokalemia, infection, kidney failure, pain, thrombocytopenia, abdominal pain, anemia, bilirubinemia, gastrointestinal hemorrhage, leukopenia, rash, respiratory disorder, chest pain.
Pregnancy Category	B.
Drug Interactions	See »Am B isome for injection.«

Ampicillin Sodium

Brand Name	Principen.
Class of Drug	Antibiotic.
Indications	Infections due to susceptible strains of the designated micro-organisms in the following conditions: Skin and skin structure infections—caused by beta-lactamase-producing strains of *S. aureus, E. coli*, Klebsiella* spp.* (including *K. pneumoniae**), *P. mirabilis*, Bacteroides fragilis*, Enterobacter* spp.*, and *Acineto-bacter calcoaceticus**. Intra-abdominal infections—caused by beta-lactamase-producing strains of *E. coli, Klebsiella* spp. (including *K. pneumoniae**), *Bacteroides* spp. (including *B. fragilis*), and *Enterobacter* spp.* Gynecological infections—caused by beta-lactamase-producing strains of *E. coli** and *Bacteroides* spp.* (including *B. fragilis**). (*Efficacy for this organism in this organ system was studied in fewer than ten infections.)
Dosage Form	
Dose	*Oral*: Adults—three to four times 1 g. Pediatric patients—four times 60–100 mg/kg body weight. *IV*: three times 0.5–5 g as short infusion.
Contraindications	In patients with a history of hypersensitivity reactions to any of the penicillins.
Warnings	Serious and occasionally fatal hypersensitivity reactions have been reported in patients on penicillin therapy. These reactions are more likely to occur in individuals with a history of penicillin hypersensitivity and/or hypersensitivity reactions to multiple allergens. There have been reports of individuals with a history of penicillin hypersensitivity who experienced severe reactions when treated with cephalosporins. Before therapy with any penicillin, careful inquiry should be made concerning previous hypersensitivity reactions to penicillin, cephalosporins, and other allergens. If an allergic reaction occurs, ampicillin should be discontinued and the appropriate therapy instituted. Serious anaphylactoid reactions require immediate emergency treatment with epinephrine. Oxygen, i.v. steroids, and airway management, including intubation, should also be administered, as indicated. Pseudomembranous colitis has been reported with nearly all antibacterial agents, including ampicillin sodium, and has ranged in severity from mild to life-threatening. Therefore, it is important to consider this diagnosis in patients who present with diarrhea subsequent to the administration of antibacterial agents.
Adverse Reactions	Pain at i.m. injection site; pain at i.v. injection site; thrombo-phlebitis; diarrhea; rash; itching; nausea; vomiting; candidiasis; fatigue; malaise; headache; chest pain/flatulence; abdominal distension; glossitis; urine retention; dysuria; edema; facial swelling; erythema; chills; tightness in throat; substernal pain;

epistaxis and mucosal bleeding; atypical lymphocytosis; increased AST (SGOT), ALT (SGPT), alkaline phosphatase, and lactic acid dehydrogenase (LDH); decreased hemoglobin, hematocrit, red blood count (RBC), white blood count (WBC), neutrophils, lymphocytes, platelets; increased lymphocytes, monocytes, basophils, eosinophils, and platelets; decreased serum albumin and total proteins; increased BUN and creatinine; presence of red blood cells (RBCs) and hyaline casts in urine.

Pregnancy Category B.

Drug Interactions Low concentrations are excreted in human milk; therefore, caution should be exercised when administering to a nursing woman. Safety and effectiveness have been established for pediatric patients 1 year of age and older for skin and skin-structure infections only.

Anakinra

Brand Name Kineret.

Class of Drug Recombinant interleukin (IL)-1 receptor antagonist. Blocks biologic activity of IL-1 by competitively inhibiting IL-1 binding to the IL-1 type I receptor (IL-1RI).

Indications Moderate to severely active rheumatoid arthritis in patients 18 years of age or older who have not responded to one or more disease-modifying antirheumatic drugs (DMARDs).*Off-label*: uveitis.

Dosage Form Solution for s.c. injection 100 mg/0.67 ml.

Dose 100 mg/day s.c. injection (or every other day for patients with severe renal insufficiency or end-stage disease).

Contraindications In patients with a known hypersensitivity to the product or any of its components.

Warnings Serious and potentially fatal infections and sepsis have occurred. Safety in combination with TNF-blocking agents has not been established; preliminary data, however, suggest a higher incidence of serious infections, including neutropenia. This combination, therefore, should be attempted with extreme caution and only when no satisfactory alternative exists.

Adverse Reactions Leukopenia with combination immunomodulators; risk of serious infections; injection-site inflammation. Monitor CBC with differential, ALT, and AST every 2 weeks for first month then every 4–6 weeks.

Pregnancy Category B.

Drug Interactions Safety and efficacy in patients with juvenile rheumatoid arthritis (JRA) have not been established. Concurrent administration of etanercept and anakinra (an IL-1 antagonist) has been associated with an increased risk of serious infections and increased risk of neutropenia.

Antazoline Phosphate

Brand Name	Vasocon-A.
Class of Drug	Antihistamine, sympathomimetic (decongestant).
Indications	Temporary relief of minor symptoms of ocular pruritus/erythema caused by pollen/animal hair.
Dosage Form	Topical ophthalmic drops: antazoline 0.5%; naphazoline HCl 0.05%.
Dose	1–2 drops four times per day, as needed for symptoms.
Contraindications	In patients with heart disease, hypertension, or narrow anterior chamber angle. Not for use in children younger than 6 years of age.
Warnings	Do not use if solution has changed color or become cloudy.
Adverse Reactions	Transient burning and stinging in some; overuse may result in increased ocular redness.
Pregnancy Category	Unspecified.

Apraclonidine HCl

Brand Name	Iopidine.
Class of Drug	Glaucoma. Alpha-2 adrenergic agonist.
Indications	Short-term adjunctive therapy for intraocular pressure (IOP) reduction; control or prevent postsurgical elevations in IOP that occur in patients after argon laser trabeculoplasty, argon laser iridotomy, or Nd:YAG posterior capsulotomy. The IOP-lowering efficacy diminishes over time in some patients. This loss of effect, or tachyphylaxis, appears to be an individual occurrence with a variable time of onset and should be closely monitored. The benefit for most patients is less than 1 month.
Dosage Form	Topical ophthalmic solution 0.5%.
Dose	One drop two to three times per day.
Contraindications	In patients receiving monoamine oxidase inhibitor (MAOI) therapy or patients with hypersensitivity to the product or any of its components or to clonidine.
Warnings	Caution should be observed in treating patients with severe, uncontrolled cardiovascular disease, hypertension, coronary insufficiency, recent myocardial infarction, renal impairment, impaired liver function, Raynaud's disease, or thromboangiitis obliterans. May decrease mental alertness.
Adverse Reactions	*Ocular*: Hyperemia (13%), pruritus (10%), discomfort (6%), tearing (4%). Reported in less than 3% of the patients—lid edema, blurred vision, foreign-body sensation, dry eye, con-

junctivitis, discharge, blanching. Reported in less than 1% of patients—lid-margin crusting, conjunctival follicles, conjunctival edema, edema, abnormal vision, pain, lid disorder, keratitis, blepharitis, photophobia, corneal staining, lid erythema, blepharoconjunctivitis, irritation, corneal erosion, corneal infiltrate, keratopathy, lid scales, lid retraction. *Nonocular:* Body as a whole—reported in less than 3% of patients: headache, asthenia; reported in less than 1% of patients: chest pain, abnormal coordination, malaise, facial edema. Cardiovascular—reported in less than 1% of patients: peripheral edema, arrhythmia; although no reports of bradycardia were available from clinical studies, the possibility of its occurrence based on apraclonidine's alpha-2-agonist effect should be considered. CNS—reported in less than 1% of patients: somnolence, dizziness, nervousness, depression, insomnia, paresthesia. Digestive system—dry mouth (10%); reported in less than 1% of the patients: constipation, nausea. Musculoskeletal—myalgia (0.2%). Respiratory system—dry nose (2%); reported in less than 1% of the patients: rhinitis, dyspnea, pharyngitis, asthma. Skin—reported in less than 1% of the patients: contact dermatitis, dermatitis. Special senses—taste perversion (3%), parosmia (0.2%).

Pregnancy Category C.

Drug Interactions Should not be used in patients receiving MAOIs (see »Contraindications«). Although no specific drug interactions with topical glaucoma drugs or systemic medications were identified in clinical studies, the possibility of an additive or potentiating effect with CNS depressants (alcohol, barbiturates, opiates, sedatives, anesthetics) should be considered. Tricyclic antidepressants (TCAs) have been reported to blunt the hypotensive effect of systemic clonidine. It is not known whether the concurrent use of these agents with apraclonidine can lead to a reduction in IOP-lowering effect. No data on the level of circulating catecholamines after apraclonidine withdrawal are available. Caution, however, is advised in patients taking TCAs, which can affect the metabolism and uptake of circulating amines. An additive hypotensive effect has been reported with the combination of systemic clonidine and neuroleptic therapy. Systemic clonidine may inhibit the production of catecholamines in response to insulin-induced hypoglycemia and mask the signs and symptoms of hypoglycemia. Since apraclonidine may reduce pulse and blood pressure, caution in using drugs such as beta-blockers (ophthalmic and systemic), antihypertensives, and cardiac glycosides is advised. Patients using cardiovascular drugs concurrently with apraclonidine 0.5% ophthalmic solution should have pulse and blood pressures frequently monitored. Caution should be exercised with simultaneous use of clonidine and other similar pharmacologic agents.

Atropine

Brand Name	Atropine-Care; Atrosulf-1; Isopto Atropine.
Class of Drug	Anticholinergic (a naturally occurring alkaloid of the belladonna plant).
Indications	Mydriatic and cycloplegic (anticholinergic). Anterior uveitis (although prolonged action may not be desirable in acute cases with self-limited course); postoperatively to provide cycloplegia after retina/vitreous and glaucoma surgery; cycloplegic refraction in children.
Dosage Form	*Topical ophthalmic solution*: 0.5%, 1%. *Topical ophthalmic ointment* 0.5%, 1%.
Dose	1 drop up to four times per day
Contraindications	In most angle-closure situations, infants, albinos, and Down syndrome patients.
Warnings	Excessive use in children and certain susceptible individuals may produce general toxic symptoms. In case of severe reactions manifested by hypotension with progressive respiratory depression, parenteral administration of physostigmine as antidote may be indicated (physostigmine 1–4 mg i.v., repeating 0.5–1.0 mg i.v. every 15 min until symptoms improve). Patient should be advised not to drive or engage in other hazardous activities while pupils are dilated.
Adverse Reactions	General signs and symptoms of atropine toxicity include dryness of mouth and skin, fever, irritability or delirium, tachycardia, and flushing of the face. Should overdosage in the eye(s) occur, flush the eye(s) with water or normal saline. Use of a topical miotic may be required. If accidentally ingested, induce emesis or gastric lavage with 4% tannic acid; 5 mg of pilocarpine should be administered orally at repeated intervals until the mouth is moist. General supportive measures should be used if needed, as listed below:*Respiratory depression*: oxygen and artificial respiration. *Urinary retention*: catheterization. *Fever*: alcohol sponge baths. Use extreme caution when employing short-acting barbiturates to control excitement. Prolonged use may produce local irritation characterized by follicular conjunctivitis, vascular congestion, edema, and exudative and eczematoid dermatitis.
Pregnancy Category	C.
Drug Interaction	As a result of atropine's effects on gastrointestinal motility and gastric emptying, absorption of other oral medications may be decreased.

Azathioprine

Brand Name	Imuran.
Class of Drug	Prodrug of 6-mercaptopurine. Antimetabolite, purine analogue. Competitively inhibits purine synthesis, blocks DNA replication and RNA synthesis. Suppresses both B and T lymphocytes.
Indications	Organ transplant surgery, dermatologic and autoimmune diseases, rheumatoid arthritis. *Ophthalmic*: treatment of various corticosteroid-resistant ocular inflammatory diseases and uveitic syndromes; scleritis associated with relapsing polychondritis; as an adjunctive, second-line agent in the control of progressive conjunctival inflammation in ocular cicatricial pemphigoid; JRA-associated iridocyclitis nonresponsive to conventional steroid therapy; Adamantiades–Behçet disease; multifocal choroiditis with panuveitis; sympathetic ophthalmia; Vogt–Koyanagi–Harada syndrome (VKH); sarcoidosis; pars planitis; Reiter's-syndrome-associated iridocyclitis.
Dosage Form	*Oral*: tablets 50 mg. *IV*: lyophilized powder equivalent to 100 mg of drug.
Dose	A single or divided oral dose administered as 2–3 mg/kg per day. Monitor CBC with differential, ALT, and AST every 2 weeks for the first month then every 4–6 weeks.
Contraindications	In patients with a history of hypersensitivity to the drug or in those who are immunosuppressed. Avoid whenever possible in pregnant women, as the drug has been shown to cross the placenta in humans. Not recommended in nursing mothers. Patients with rheumatoid arthritis previously treated with alkylating agents (cyclophosphamide, chlorambucil, melphalan, or others) may have a prohibitive risk of neoplasia if treated with azathioprine.
Warnings	Chronic immunosuppression with this purine antimetabolite may increase risk of neoplasia in humans. Severe leukopenia and/or thrombocytopenia may occur.
Adverse Reactions	*Bone marrow suppression*: with leukopenia and thrombocytopenia are common, dose dependent, and may occur late in the course of therapy. Dose reduction or temporary withdrawal allows reversal of these toxicities. Myelosuppression is delayed (appearing 1–2 weeks after initiation of therapy). *Neoplasia*: increased risk of malignancies (non-Hodgkin lymphoma). *Gastrointestinal*: GI discomfort, anorexia, nausea, vomiting, and diarrhea are the most common. Others include hepatocellular necrosis, pancreatitis, stomatitis, and steatorrhea. A rare but life-threatening hepatic venoocclusive disease associated with chronic administration of azathioprine has been described. *Others*: rash, alopecia, fever, arthralgias, negative nitrogen balance, interstitial pneumonitis, secondary infections.

Pregnancy Category   D.
Drug Interactions   Inhibits xanthine oxidase, thereby impairing conversion of azathioprine to its metabolites. Dosage should therefore be reduced by 25% in patients treated concomitantly with these medications. Drugs that may affect leukocyte production, including cotrimoxazole, may lead to exaggerated leukopenia, especially in renal transplant recipients. The use of angiotensin-converting enzyme inhibitors to control hypertension in patients on azathioprine has been reported to induce severe leukopenia. May inhibit the anticoagulant effect of warfarin. Clearance may be affected by drugs that inhibit (ketoconazole, erythromycin) or induce (phenantoin, rifampin, phenobarbital) the hepatic microsomal enzyme system.

Azelastine

Brand Name   Optivar.
Class of Drug   Selective histamine H1 antagonist.
Indications   Itching of the eye associated with allergic conjunctivitis.
Dosage Form   Topical ophthalmic solution 0.05%.
Dose   1 drop to affected eye two times per day
Contraindications   In patients with a known hypersensitivity to the product or any of its components.
Warnings   Ocular use only.
Adverse Reactions   Transient eye burning/stinging (~30%), headaches (~15%), bitter taste (~10%). The following have been reported in 1–10% of patients: asthma, conjunctivitis, dyspnea, eye pain, fatigue, influenza-like symptoms, pharyngitis, pruritus, rhinitis, temporary blurring.
Pregnancy Category   C.
Drug Interactions   Caution should be exercised in nursing mothers. Safety and effectiveness in patients younger than 3 years of age has not been established.

Bacitracin Zinc

Class of Drug	Antibiotic. Interferes with bacterial cell-wall synthesis.
Indications	Topical treatment of superficial infections of external eye; adnexa, such as conjunctivitis, keratitis, keratoconjunctivitis, blepharitis, and blepharoconjunctivitis; active against most gram-positive bacilli/cocci, including hemolytic streptococci.
Dosage Form	Topical ophthalmic ointment 500 U/g.
Dose	Apply small amount of ointment to affected eye(s) every 3–4 h for 7–10 days based on severity of infection.
Contraindications	In patients with a known hypersensitivity to the product or any of its components. Contact lenses should not be used with redness in eye. Soft lenses should not be placed in non-red eye for at least 10 min after application.
Warnings	*Not for injection into the eye.* Topical antibiotics may cause cutaneous sensitization. Manifestations of sensitization include itching, reddening, and edema of conjunctiva and eyelid.
Adverse Reactions	Tend to be allergic sensitizations, including itching, swelling, and conjunctival erythema; exact incidence unknown. Serious hypersensitivity reactions, including anaphylaxis, have been rarely reported.
Pregnancy Category	C.
Brand Name	Cortisporin. (bacitracin zinc, hydrocortisone, neomycin, polymyxin B sulfates).
Class of Drug	Antibiotic/corticosteroid combination.
Indications	Activity as with Polysporin whenever a combination of antibiotics and steroids is indicated.
Dosage Form	Topical ophthalmic ointment: each gram contains 400 U bacitracin, hydrocortisone 1%, 3.5 mg neomycin, and 10,000 U polymyxin B.
Dose	Apply small amount of ointment to affected eye(s) every 3–4 h for 7–10 days based on severity of infection. If used beyond 10 days, see »Warnings« and »Adverse Reactions.«
Contraindications	In most viral diseases of the cornea and conjunctiva, including epithelial herpes simplex keratitis (dendritic keratitis), vaccinia, and varicella, and also in mycobacterial infection of the eye and fungal diseases of ocular structures. Also in patients who have shown hypersensitivity to the product or any of its components. Hypersensitivity to the antibiotic component occurs at a higher rate than for other components.
Warnings	Prolonged use of corticosteroids may result in ocular hypertension and/or glaucoma with damage to the optic nerve, defects in visual acuity and fields of vision, and posterior subcapsular cataract formation. Prolonged use may suppress the host response and thus increase the hazard of secondary ocular infections. In those diseases causing thinning of the cornea

or sclera, perforations have been known to occur with the use of topical corticosteroids. In acute purulent conditions of the eye, corticosteroids may mask infection or enhance existing infection. If these products are used for 10 days or longer, IOP should be routinely monitored even though it may be difficult in uncooperative patients. Corticosteroids should be used with caution in the presence of glaucoma. Use of ocular corticosteroids may prolong the course and may exacerbate the severity of many viral infections of the eye (including herpes simplex). Employment of corticosteroid medication in the treatment of herpes simplex requires great caution.

Adverse Reactions
Due to the corticosteroid component in decreasing order of frequency: elevation of IOP with possible development of glaucoma and infrequent optic nerve damage, posterior subcapsular cataract formation, and delayed wound healing.

Secondary infection: Has occurred after use of combinations containing corticosteroids and antimicrobials. Fungal and viral infections of the cornea are particularly prone to develop coincidentally with long-term applications of a corticosteroid. The possibility of fungal invasion must be considered in any persistent corneal ulceration where corticosteroid treatment has been used. Local irritation on instillation has been reported.

Pregnancy Category
C.

Drug Interactions
See »Neosporin.«

Brand Name
Neosporin (neomycin and polymyxin B sulfates and bacitracin zinc).

Class of Drug
Antibiotic.*Neomycin*: inhibits protein synthesis by binding with ribosomal RNA. *Polymyxin B*: increases permeability of bacterial cell membrane.

Indications
Topical treatment of superficial infections of external eye; adnexa such as conjunctivitis, keratitis, keratoconjunctivitis, blepharitis, blepharoconjunctivitis; along with polymyxin B sulfate and neomycin, considered active against *S. aureus*; streptococci, including *Streptococcus pneumoniae*; *E. coli*; *Haemophilus influenzae*; *Klebsiella/Enterobacter* spp.; *Neisseria* spp.; and *P. aeruginosa*; not adequate coverage against *Serratia marcescens*.

Dosage Form
Topical ophthalmic ointment: each gram contains neomycin sulfate equivalent to 3.5 mg neomycin base, polymyxin B sulfate equivalent to 10,000 U polymyxin B, and bacitracin zinc equivalent to 400 U bacitracin.

Dose
Apply a small amount of ointment to the affected eye(s) every 3–4 h for 7–10 days based on severity of infection.

Contraindications
In patients with a known hypersensitivity to the product or any of its components. Contact lenses should not be used with redness in eye. Soft lenses should not be placed in non-red eye for at least 10 min after application.

Warnings	*Not for injection into the eye.* Topical antibiotics may cause cutaneous sensitization. Manifestations of sensitization include itching, reddening, and edema of conjunctiva and eyelid.
Adverse Reactions	Tend to be allergic sensitizations, including itching, swelling, and conjunctival erythema; exact incidence unknown. Serious hypersensitivity reactions, including anaphylaxis, have been rarely reported.
Pregnancy Category	C.
Drug Interactions	Allergic cross-reactions may occur with the following, which may prevent their use: kanamycin, paromomycin, streptomycin, and gentamicin (possible). Long-term studies in animals to determine carcinogenesis have not been conducted. Since there are no adequate controlled studies in pregnant women, this drug should be used only when clearly needed.

Brand Name	Polysporin (bacitracin zinc and polymyxin B sulfate).
Class of Drug	Antibiotic.
Indications	Superficial ocular infections involving conjunctiva or cornea. *Bacitracin*: active against most gram-positive bacilli/cocci, including hemolytic streptococci. *Polymyxin B*: active against gram-negative bacilli (including *P. aeruginosa, H. influenza*).
Dosage Form	Topical ophthalmic ointment: each gram contains 500 U bacitracin and 10,000 U polymyxin B sulfate.
Dose	Apply a small amount of ointment to affected eye(s) every 3–4 h for 7–10 days based on severity of infection.
Contraindications	In patients with a known hypersensitivity to the product or any of its components.
Warnings	Ophthalmic ointments may inhibit corneal healing.
Adverse Reactions	See »Neosporin.«
Pregnancy Category	C.
Drug Interactions	See »Neosporin.«

Betaxolol

Brand Name	Betoptic S.
Class of Drug	Glaucoma. Selective beta-adrenergic-blocking agents.
Indications	Decrease IOP in chronic OAG and ocular hypertension.
Dosage Form	Topical ophthalmic suspension 0.25%.
Dose	1–2 drops to affected eye(s) two times per day
Contraindications	In patients with a known hypersensitivity to the product or any of its components. In patients with sinus bradycardia, more than first-degree AV (AV) block, cardiogenic shock, or overt cardiac failure.
Warnings	*Cardiac/respiratory*: Topical application may result in systemic absorption. Same adverse reactions in topical adminis-

tration as in systemic administration: severe cardiac/respiratory reactions (including death due to bronchospasm) and, rarely, death due to heart failure. Caution in patients with heart block or heart failure. *Diabetes mellitus*: caution in patients subject to hypoglycemic episodes since beta-blocking drugs may mask symptoms of acute hypoglycemia. *Thyrotoxicosis*: beta-blockers may mask clinical signs, such as tachycardia; abrupt withdrawal of beta-blockers in suspected patients should be avoided since it might precipitate thyroid storm. *Myasthenia*: beta-adrenergic blockade may potentiate muscle weakness symptoms (diplopia, ptosis, generalized weakness). *Major surgery*: consideration given to gradual withdrawal of beta-adrenergic agents prior to general anesthesia because of reduced ability of heart to respond to reflex sympathetic stimuli. *Pulmonary*: asthmatic attacks and respiratory distress during betaxolol treatment have been reported.

Adverse Reactions
Most frequent: transient ocular discomfort. *Reported in small number of patients*: blurred vision, corneal punctate keratitis, foreign-body sensation, photophobia, tearing, itching, dryness, ocular pain, decreased visual acuity, and crusty lashes. *Systemic*: have been rarely reported.

Pregnancy Category
C.

Drug Interactions
There are no adequate and well-controlled studies in pregnant women. It should be used only when benefit justifies potential risk to fetus. Long-term studies in animals demonstrate no carcinogenic effect. In vivo/in vitro tests did not demonstrate mutagenicity. Patients receiving a beta-adrenergic agent orally and betaxolol ophthalmically should be observed for potential additive effects. Patients should also be closely monitored when receiving catecholamine-depleting drugs, such as reserpine, because of additive effects and hypotension/bradycardia. Caution should be exercised in nursing mothers. Safety and effectiveness in pediatric population is not established.

Bimatoprost

Brand Name
Lumigan.

Class of Drug
Prostaglandin hypotensive.

Indications
IOP reduction in OAG or ocular hypertension in patients who are refractory or intolerant to other medication.

Dosage Form
Topical ophthalmic solution 0.03%.

Dose
1 drop to affected eye(s) once per day in the evenings. Should not be used more than once per day.

Contraindications	In patients with a known hypersensitivity to the product or any of its components exist.
Warnings	Reported to cause changes to pigmented tissues (increased pigmentation), growth of eyelashes, increased pigmentation of iris and periorbital tissues; changes may be permanent. Patients should be informed of the possibility of iris color change. Should be used with caution in patients with active ocular inflammation. Macular edema, including cystoid macular edema, has been reported during treatment. Should be used with caution in patients with a torn posterior lens capsule, aphakic or pseudophakic patients, and patients with macular edema risk factors. May be associated with recurrence of Herpes simplex keratitis.
Adverse Reactions	Conjunctival hyperemia, growth of eyelashes, and ocular pruritus (15–45% of patients); ocular dryness, visual disturbance, foreign-body sensation, eye pain, skin pigmentation or periocular skin, blepharitis, cataract, superficial punctate keratopathy, eyelid erythema (3–10% of patients); eye discharge, tearing, photophobia, allergic conjunctivitis, asthenopia, increase of pigmentation, conjunctival edema (1–3% of patients); iritis was reported in more than 1% of patients. *Systemic*: infections, mostly colds; upper respiratory tract infections (URTIs) (~10% of patients); headaches, abnormal LFTs, asthenia, hirsutism (1–5% of patients).
Pregnancy Category	C.
Drug Interactions	There are no adequate and well-controlled studies in pregnant women. It should be used only when benefit justifies potential risk to the fetus. Caution should be exercised in nursing mothers. Safety and effectiveness in the pediatric population is not established.

Boric Acid

Brand Name	Collyrium Fresh Eyes.
Class of Drug	Eye wash.
Indications	Cleanse the eye and remove loose foreign material, air pollutants, etc.
Dosage Form	Solution.
Dose	Flush affected eye as needed.
Warnings	Discontinue if change in vision or eye pain occur, if redness or irritation persist, or if condition worsens or persists.
Pregnancy Category	C.
Brand Name	Eye Wash Solution.
Class of Drug	Eye wash.

Indications	See »Collyrium Fresh Eyes.«
Dosage Form	See »Collyrium Fresh Eyes.«
Dose	See »Collyrium Fresh Eyes.«
Warnings	See »Collyrium Fresh Eyes.«
Pregnancy Category	C.

Brimonidine

Brand Name	Alphagan.
Class of Drug	Glaucoma. Alpha-2 adrenergic agonist.
Indications	OAG; ocular hypertension.
Dosage Form	Topical ophthalmic solution 0.2% (benzalkonium chloride preservative).
Dose	1 drop to affected eye(s) three times per day The IOP-lowering effect diminishes over time in some patients. This loss of effect appears with a variable time of onset in each patient and should be closely monitored.
Contraindications	In patients receiving MAOIs or in patients with a known hypersensitivity to the product or any of its components. Caution to be exercised in those with severe cardiovascular disease, hepatic/renal impairment, depression, coronary or cerebral insufficiency, Raynaud's phenomenon, orthostatic hypotension, thromboangiitis obliterans. May cause drowsiness and/or fatigue; caution to be exercised during hazardous activities.
Warnings	Agitation, apnea, bradycardia, convulsion, cyanosis, depression, dyspnea, emotional instabilities, hypotension, hypothermia, hypotonia, hypoventilation, irritability, lethargy, somnolence, and stupor have been reported in pediatric patients.
Adverse Reactions	In descending order of incidence: oral dryness, ocular hyperemia, burning and stinging, headache, blurring, foreign-body sensation, fatigue/drowsiness, conjunctival follicles, ocular allergic reactions, and ocular pruritus (10–30% of patients); corneal staining/erosion, photophobia, eyelid erythema, ocular ache/pain, ocular dryness, tearing, upper respiratory symptoms, eyelid edema, conjunctival edema, dizziness, blepharitis, ocular irritation, gastrointestinal symptoms, asthenia, conjunctival blanching, abnormal vision, and muscular pains (3–9% of patients); lid crusting, conjunctival hemorrhage, abnormal taste, insomnia, conjunctival discharge, depression, hypertension, anxiety, palpitations/arrhythmias, nasal dryness and syncope (less than 3% of patients).*Postmarketing use*: bradycardia, hypotension, iritis, miosis, skin reactions, tachycardia (frequency unknown). In infants, apnea, bradycardia, hypotension, hypotonia, and somnolence have been reported.

Pregnancy Category	B.
Drug Interactions	No carcinogenic, mutagenic, or impairment of fertility noted in animal studies. No specific drug interaction studies have been conducted. May cause additive effects with CNS depressants. Use caution with beta-blockers, antihypertensives, cardiac glycosides, TCAs. In animal studies, brimonidine tartrate was excreted in human milk. Not recommended in children younger than 2 years of age.

Brand Name	Alphagan-P.
Class of Drug	See »Alphagan.«
Indications	See »Alphagan.«
Dosage Form	Topical ophthalmic solution 0.15% (purite preservative).
Dose	See »Alphagan.«
Contraindications	See »Alphagan.«
Warnings	See »Alphagan.«
Adverse Reactions	Allergic conjunctivitis, conjunctival hyperemia, ocular pruritus (10–20% of patients); burning sensation, conjunctival folliculosis, hypertension, oral dryness, visual disturbance (~5–9% of patients); allergic reaction, asthenia, blepharitis, bronchitis, conjunctival edema, conjunctival hemorrhage, conjunctivitis, cough, dizziness, dyspepsia, dyspnea, epiphora, eye discharge, eye dryness, eye irritation, eye pain, eyelid edema, eyelid erythema, flu-like symptoms, follicular conjunctivitis, foreign-body sensation, headache, pharyngitis, photophobia, rash, rhinitis, sinus infection, sinusitis, stinging, superficial punctate keratitis (SPK), visual-field defect, vitreous floaters, decreased visual acuity (~1–4% of patients). Postmarketing experience: see »Alphagan.«
Pregnancy Category	B.
Drug Interactions	See »Alphagan.«

Brinzolamide

Brand Name	Azopt.
Class of Drug	Glaucoma. CAI.
Indications	OAG; ocular hypertension.
Dosage Form	Topical ophthalmic suspension 1%.
Dose	1 drop to affected eye(s) three times per day
Contraindications	In patients who are hypersensitive to the product or any of its components.
Warnings	Same types of adverse reactions attributable to sulfonamides may occur with topical administration (see »Warnings« under acetazolamide). If signs of serious reactions or hypersensitivity occur, discontinue use. The effect of continued ad-

ministration on the corneal endothelium has not been fully evaluated. Has not been studied in patients with acute ACG. Because Azopt and its metabolite are excreted predominantly by the kidney, it is not recommended in patients with severe renal impairment. Has not been studied in patients with hepatic impairment and should be used with caution in such patients. Since there is a potential for an additive effect, concomitant administration with oral carbonic anhydrase inhibitors is not recommended.

Adverse Reactions *Most frequent*: blurred vision and bitter, sour, or unusual taste (approximately 5–10% of patients); blepharitis, dermatitis, dry eye, foreign-body sensation, headache, hyperemia, ocular discharge, ocular discomfort, ocular keratitis, ocular pain, ocular pruritus, and rhinitis (1–5% of patients); allergic reactions, alopecia, chest pain, conjunctivitis, diarrhea, diplopia, dizziness, dry mouth, dyspnea, dyspepsia, eye fatigue, hypertonia, keratoconjunctivitis, keratopathy, kidney pain, lid-margin crusting or sticky sensation, nausea, pharyngitis, tearing, urticaria (less than 1% of patients).

Pregnancy Category C.

Drug Interactions Carcinogenicity data are not available. Most tests for mutagenic potential were negative (except in in vitro mouse lymphoma forward mutation assay with microsomal activation). In reproduction studies in rats, there were no adverse effects on the fertility or reproduction. Because many drugs are excreted in human milk, and because of the potential for serious adverse reactions, a decision should be made whether to discontinue nursing or to discontinue the drug, taking into account the importance of the drug to the mother. Safety and effectiveness in pediatric patients have not been established. Rare instances of drug interactions have occurred with high-dose salicylate therapy; therefore, the potential for such drug interactions should be considered.

Bromocriptine

Brand Name Parlodel.

Class of Drug Semisynthetic ergot alkaloid as an inhibitor of prolactin secretion. Shown to stimulate directly and compete with specific binding to dopaminergic receptors in various tissues throughout the body. Inhibitor of prolactin secretion (prolactin has powerful immunomodulatory properties).

Indications Parkinson's disease; conditions associated with hyperprolactinemia, including amenorrhea and galactorrhea; female infertility; postpartum lactation; pituitary adenoma; adjunctive agent in management of noninfectious ocular inflammation disease; effective in the treatment of thyroid ophthalmopathy.

Dosage Form	Oral:*capsules* 5 mg; *tablets* 2.5 mg.
Dose	1.25 mg with food at bedtime gradually increased to 2.5 mg three or four times per day
Contraindications	In patients with uncontrolled systemic hypertension, toxemia of pregnancy, or a history of hypersensitivity to ergot alkaloids.
Warnings	Crosses the placenta and may suppress fetal prolactin levels; should be avoided during pregnancy unless indicated. Mothers who choose to breast-feed their infants should avoid bromocriptine since it suppresses lactation. Caution must be exercised in administering concurrently with any antihypertensive medication.
Adverse Reactions	Nausea, vomiting, postural hypotension, headache, dyspepsia, constipation, nasal congestion, dryness of the mouth, nocturnal leg cramps, depression, impaired concentration, nightmares, peripheral digital vasospasm on exposure to cold, pleural thickening, dry eye.
Drug Interactions	Hepatic clearance may be reduced by concomitant administration of erythromycin. Efficacy may be diminished in patients who are also receiving agents that exhibit clopamine antagonism (i.e., phenothiazines).
Pregnancy Category	B.

Bupivacaine

Brand Name	Marcaine; Sensorcaine.
Class of Drug	Local anesthetic.
Indications	Local anesthesia for surgery; major nerve block for surgery.
Dosage Form	Parenteral for injection 0.25, 0.5, 0.75%; maximum dose 150 mg.
Dose	Maximum dose 2 mg/kg body weight. Slow onset (10–20 min), lasts for 4–8 h.
Contraindications	*Most significant*: infection at site. *Significant*: disease of cardiovascular system, myasthenia gravis, plasma cholinesterase deficiency. *Possibly significant*: diseases of liver, renal disease.
Adverse Reactions	Allergic reactions, anaphylaxis, cardiac arrhythmias, CNS toxicity, erythema, methemoglobinemia, myocardial dysfunction, nausea, pruritus, skin rash, sneezing, urticaria, vasodilation of blood vessels, vomiting.
Drug Interactions	Possibly safe in pregnancy. It is not known whether this drug or its metabolites are excreted in human milk. Safety and effectiveness in pediatric patients have not been established.

Warnings   The 0.75% solution not be used in patients in late pregnan-
                          cy. It was also recommended always to inject in incremental
                          doses while closely observing for signs of accidental i.v. injec-
                          tion.
Pregnancy Category   B.

Carbachol

Brand Name
Carbastat; Miostat.

Class of Drug
Surgery, ophthalmic, adjunct, parasympathomimetic, miotic, dual action; direct cholinergic as well as partial inhibitor of cholinesterase.

Indications
Intraoperative miosis as well as reducing intensity of IOP spike in the first 24 h.

Dosage Form
Sterile, balanced, salt solution of carbachol for intraocular injection 0.01%.

Dose
Solution for injection 0.01% .

Contraindications
Carbachol intraocular injection: in patients showing hypersensitivity to the product or any of its components.

Warnings
For single-dose intraocular use only. Discard unused portion. Intraocular carbachol 0.01% should be used with caution in patients with acute cardiac failure, bronchial asthma, peptic ulcer, hyperthyroidism, GI spasm, urinary tract obstruction, and Parkinson's disease.

Adverse Reactions
Systemic side effects, such as flushing, sweating, epigastric distress, abdominal cramps, tightness in urinary bladder, and headache have been reported with topical or systemic application.

Pregnancy Category
C.

Brand Name
Isopto Carbachol; Carboptic.

Class of Drug
Parasympathomimetic, miotic, dual action. Direct cholinergic as well as partial inhibitor of cholinesterase.

Indications
Glaucoma.

Dosage Form
Topical ophthalmic solution 0.75%, 1.5%, 2.25%, 3.0%.

Dose
1–2 drops up to three times per day

Contraindications
Miotics are contraindicated where constriction is undesirable, such as acute iritis or in patients showing hypersensitivity to the product or any of its components.

Warnings
Should be used with caution in the presence of corneal abrasion to avoid excessive penetration, which can produce systemic toxicity, and in patients with acute cardiac failure, bronchial asthma, active peptic ulcer, hyperthyroidism, gastrointestinal spasm, urinary tract obstruction, Parkinson's disease, recent myocardial infarct, systemic hypertension or hypotension. As with all miotics, retinal detachment has been reported when used in certain susceptible individuals. Remove contact lenses before using.

Adverse Reactions
Transient symptoms of stinging and burning may occur. Capable of producing systemic symptoms of cholinesterase inhibitor, even when epithelium is intact. Transient ciliary and conjunctival injection, headache, and ciliary spasm with resultant temporary decrease of visual acuity may occur. Salivation, syncope, cardiac arrhythmia, gastrointestinal cramping, vomiting, asthma, hypotension, diarrhea, frequent urge to urinate, increased sweating, and eye irritation may occur.

Pregnancy Category
C.

Carboxymethyl-cellulose

Brand Name	Refresh Celluvisc.
Class of Drug	Lubricant eye drops.
Indications	Temporary relief of burning, irritation, and discomfort due to eye dryness or exposure to wind or sun; may be used as a protectant against further irritation.
Dosage Form	Topical ophthalmic solution. Carboxymethyl-cellulose sodium 1%. Preservative free.
Dose	1 or 2 drops to affected eye(s) as needed; discard container.
Pregnancy Category	C.

Brand Name	Refresh Liquigel.
Class of Drug	Lubricant eye drops.
Indications	See »Refresh Celluvisc.«
Dosage Form	Topical ophthalmic solution. Carboxymethyl-cellulose sodium 1%.
Dose	1 or 2 drops to affected eye(s) as needed.
Pregnancy Category	C.

Brand Name	Refresh Plus.
Class of Drug	Lubricant eye drops.
Indications	See »Refresh Celluvisc.«
Dosage Form	Topical ophthalmic solution. Carboxymethyl-cellulose sodium 0.5%. Preservative free.
Dose	1 or 2 drops to affected eye(s) as needed, and discard container.
Pregnancy Category	C.

Brand Name	Refresh Tears.
Class of Drug	Lubricant eye drops.
Indications	See »Refresh Celluvisc.«
Dosage Form	Topical ophthalmic solution. Carboxymethyl-cellulose sodium 0.5%.
Dose	1 or 2 drops to affected eye(s) as needed.
Pregnancy Category	C.

Carteolol Hydrochloride

Brand Name	Ocupress.
Class of Drug	Glaucoma. Nonselective beta-adrenergic blocker.
Indications	Lowering IOP in chronic OAG and intraocular hypertension.

Dosage Form   Topical ophthalmic solution 1%.

Dose   1 drop to affected eye(s) two times per day

Contraindications   In patients with bronchial asthma or with a history of bronchial asthma or severe chronic obstructive pulmonary disease (see »Warnings«), sinus bradycardia, second- and third-degree AV block, overt cardiac failure (see »Warnings«), cardiogenic shock, or hypersensitivity to the product or any of its components.

Warnings   The same adverse reactions found with systemic administration of beta-adrenergic-blocking agents may occur with topical administration. Severe respiratory reactions and cardiac reactions, including death due to bronchospasm, in patients with asthma and, rarely, death in association with cardiac failure have been reported with topical application of beta-adrenergic-blocking agents. *Cardiac failure*: In patients without a history of cardiac failure, continued depression of the myocardium with beta-blocking agents over a period of time can, in some cases, lead to cardiac failure. At the first sign or symptom of cardiac failure, carteolol hydrochloride should be discontinued. *Nonallergic bronchospasm*: in patients with nonallergic bronchospasm or with a history of nonallergic bronchospasm carteolol, should be administered with caution since it may block bronchodilation produced by endogenous and exogenous catecholamine stimulation of beta 2 receptors. *Major surgery*: The necessity of withdrawal of beta-adrenergic-blocking agents prior to major surgery is controversial. Beta-adrenergic receptor blockade may impair the ability of the heart to respond to beta-adrenergically mediated reflex stimuli, augment the risk of general anesthesia, or result in protracted severe hypotension during anesthesia. For these reasons, in patients undergoing elective surgery, gradual withdrawal of beta-adrenergic-blocking agents may be appropriate. If necessary, during surgery, the effects of beta-adrenergic-blocking agents may be reversed by sufficient doses of such agonists as isoproterenol, dopamine, dobutamine, or levarterenol. *Diabetes mellitus*: Beta-adrenergic-blocking agents should be administered with caution in patients subject to spontaneous hypoglycemia or diabetic patients (especially those with labile diabetes). May also mask the signs and symptoms of acute hypoglycemia. *Thyrotoxicosis*: Beta-adrenergic-blocking agents may mask certain clinical signs (e.g., tachycardia) of hyperthyroidism. Patients suspected of developing thyrotoxicosis should be managed carefully to avoid abrupt withdrawal of beta-adrenergic-blocking agents, which might precipitate a thyroid storm. *Muscle weakness*: beta-adrenergic blockade has been reported to potentiate muscle weakness consistent with certain myasthenic symptoms (e.g., diplopia, ptosis, and generalized weakness).

Adverse Reactions   *Ocular*: transient eye irritation, burning, tearing, and conjunctival hyperemia and edema occurred in about one of four patients; other ocular symptoms, including blurred and cloudy vision, photophobia, decreased night vision, and ptosis and ocular signs, including blepharoconjunctivitis, abnormal corneal staining, and corneal sensitivity, occurred occasionally. *Systemic*: As is characteristic of nonselective adrenergic blocking agents, may cause bradycardia and decreased blood pressure (see »Warnings«). The following systemic events have occasionally been reported: cardiac arrhythmia, heart palpitation, dyspnea, asthenia, headache, dizziness, insomnia, sinusitis, and taste perversion. The following additional adverse reactions have been reported with ophthalmic use of beta-1 and beta-2 (nonselective) adrenergic-receptor-blocking agents: Body as a whole—headache. Cardiovascular—arrhythmia, syncope, heart block, cerebral vascular accident, cerebral ischemia, congestive heart failure, palpitations (see »Warnings«). Digestive—nausea. Psychiatric—depression. Skin—hypersensitivity, including localized and generalized rash. Respiratory—bronchospasm (predominantly in patients with preexisting bronchospastic disease), respiratory failure (see »Warnings«). Endocrine—masked symptoms of hypoglycemia in insulin-dependent diabetics (see »Warnings«). Special senses—signs and symptoms of keratitis; blepharoptosis; visual disturbances, including refractive changes (due to withdrawal of miotic therapy in some cases); diplopia; ptosis. Other reactions associated with the oral use of nonselective adrenergic receptor blocking agents should be considered potential effects with ophthalmic use of these agents.

Pregnancy Category   C.
Drug Interactions   Did not produce carcinogenic effects at doses up to 40 mg/ kg per day in 2-year oral rat and mouse studies. Tests of mutagenicity demonstrated no evidence for mutagenic potential. Should be used with caution in patients receiving a beta-adrenergic-blocking agent orally because of the potential for additive effects on systemic beta blockade. Close observation is recommended when a beta-blocker is administered to patients receiving catecholamine-depleting drugs, such as reserpine, because of possible additive effects and the production of hypotension and/or marked bradycardia, which may produce vertigo, syncope, or postural hypotension.

Cefazolin Sodium

Brand Name   Ancef; Kefzol.

Class of Drug   Antibiotic.

Indications   Keratitis; corneal ulcer; gram-positive bacilli and cocci (except*Enterococcus*); some gram-negative bacilli, including *E. coli, Proteus* spp., and *Klebsiella* spp.

Dosage Form   IV 500 mg, 1 g.

Dose   Usual adult dose: 250 mg to 2 g every 8 h. Perioperative prophylaxis: 1 g 30–60 min prior to surgery for clean and contaminated surgery; 1 g every 8 h for dirty or traumatic surgery.

Contraindications   Increased levels with probenecid.

Warnings   Modify dosage in patients with severe renal impairment. Prolonged use may result in superinfection. Use with caution in patients with a history of penicillin allergy, especially IgE-mediated reactions.

Adverse Reactions   Diarrhea (1–10% of patients); CNS irritation, seizures, abdominal cramps, fever rash, eosinophilia, hypothrombinemia, urticaria, leucopenia, pseudomembranous colitis, transient elevation of liver enzymes, pain at injection site, superinfections, anaphylaxis, Stevens–Johnson syndrome, oral candidiasis, nausea, vomiting, anorexia, phlebitis (less than 1% of patients).

Pregnancy Category   B.

Drug Interactions   May decrease renal tubular secretion of cephalosporins when used concurrently, resulting in increased and more prolonged cephalosporin blood levels. A false positive reaction for glucose in the urine may occur with Benedict's solution, Fehling's solution, or with Clinitest tablets but not with enzyme-based tests such as Clinistix. Positive direct and indirect antiglobulin (Coombs) tests have occurred; these may also occur in neonates whose mothers received cephalosporins before delivery.

Cefotetan Disodium

Brand Name   Cefotan.

Class of Drug   Antibiotic. Cephalosporin.

Indications   Susceptible bacterial infections; less active against staphylococci and streptococci than first-generation cephalosporins but active against anaerobes, including*B. fragilis*; gram-ne-

	gative enteric bacilli, including *E. coli, Klebsiella*, and *Proteus*; mainly respiratory tract, skin and skin structures, bone and joint, intra-abdominal, urinary tract.
Dosage Form	Powder for injection 1 g, 2 g.
Dose	*Children*: i.m. and i.v. 20–40 mg/kg per dose every 12 h. *Adults*: i.m. and i.v. 1–6 g/day in divided doses every 12 h.
Contraindications	In patients who have shown hypersensitivity to cefotetan or the cephalosporin group of antibiotics.
Warnings	Modify dosage in patients with severe renal impairment; prolonged use may result in superinfection. Use with caution in patients with a history of penicillin allergy, especially IgE-mediated reactions (e.g., anaphylaxis, urticaria); may case antibiotic-associated colitis.
Adverse Reactions	Diarrhea, hypersensitivity reactions, hepatic enzyme elevation (1–10% of patients); anaphylaxis, urticaria, rash, pruritus, pseudomembranous colitis, nausea, vomiting, eosinophilia, thrombocytosis, agranulocytosis, hemolytic anemia, leucopenia, bleeding, prolonged prothrombin time (PT), elevated BUN, elevated creatinine, nephrotoxicity, phlebitis, fever (less than 1% of patients).
Pregnancy Category	B.
Drug Interactions	Increased nephrotoxicity has been reported following concomitant administration of cephalosporins and aminoglycoside antibiotics. Cephalosporins are known to occasionally induce a positive direct Coombs' test

Ceftazidime

Brand Name	Ceftaz; Fortaz; Tazicef; Tazidime.
Class of Drug	Antibiotic.
Indications	Lower respiratory infections (LRIs), including: Pneumonia—caused by *P. aeruginosa* and other *Pseudomonas* spp.; *H. influenzae*, including ampicillin-resistant strains; *Klebsiella* spp.; *Enterobacter* spp.; *Proteus mirabilis*; *E. coli*; *Serratia* spp.; *Citrobacter* spp.; *S. pneumoniae*; and *S. aureus* (methicillin-susceptible strains). Skin and skin-structure infections—caused by *P. aeruginosa*; *Klebsiella* spp.; *E. coli*; *Proteus* spp., including *P. mirabilis* and indole-positive *Proteus*; *Enterobacter* spp.; *Serratia* spp.; *S. aureus* (methicillin-susceptible strains); and *S. pyogenes* (group A beta-hemolytic streptococci). UTIs, both complicated and uncomplicated—caused by *P. aeruginosa*; *Enterobacter* spp.; *Proteus* spp., including *P. mirabilis* and indole-positive *Proteus*; *Klebsiella* spp.; and *E. coli*. Bacterial septicemia—caused by *P. aeruginosa, Klebsiella* spp., *H. influenzae*,

E. coli, Serratia spp., *S. pneumoniae*, and *S. aureus* (methicillin-susceptible strains). Bone and joint infections—caused by *P. aeruginosa, Klebsiella* spp., *Enterobacter* spp., and *S. aureus* (methicillin-susceptible strains). Gynecologic infections, including endometritis, pelvic cellulitis, and other infections of the female genital tract—caused by *E. coli*. Intra-abdominal infections, including peritonitis—caused by *E. coli, Klebsiella* spp., and *S. aureus* (methicillin-susceptible strains). Polymicrobial infections—caused by aerobic and anaerobic organisms and *Bacteroides* spp. (many strains of *B. fragilis* are resistant). CNS infections, including meningitis—caused by *H. influenzae* and *Neisseria meningitidis*. Has also been used successfully in a limited number of cases of meningitis due to *P. aeruginosa* and *S. pneumoniae*.

Dosage Form   Sterile solution for injection.

Dose   Usual adult dosage is 1 g administered i.v. or i.m. every 8–12 h. Dosage and route should be determined by susceptibility of the causative organisms, severity of infection, and condition and renal function of the patient.*Neonates (0–4 weeks)*: 30 mg/kg i.v., every 12 h. *Infants and children (1 month–12 years)*: 30–50 mg/kg i.v. to a maximum of 6 g/day, every 8 h.

Contraindications   In patients who have shown hypersensitivity to this product or any of the cephalosporin group of antibiotics.

Warnings   Before therapy is instituted, careful inquiry should be made to determine whether the patient has had previous hypersensitivity reactions to ceftazidime, cephalosporins, penicillins, or other drugs. If this product is to be given to penicillin-sensitive patients, caution should be exercised because cross-hypersensitivity among beta-lactam antibiotics has been clearly documented and may occur in up to 10% of patients with a history of penicillin allergy. If an allergic reaction occurs, discontinue the drug. Serious acute hypersensitivity reactions may require treatment with epinephrine and other emergency measures, including oxygen, i.v. fluids, i.v. antihistamines, corticosteroids, pressor amines, and airway management, as clinically indicated. Pseudomembranous colitis has been reported with nearly all antibacterial agents, including ceftazidime, and may range in severity from mild to life threatening; therefore, it is important to consider this diagnosis in patients who present with diarrhea subsequent to the administration of antibacterial agents.

Adverse Reactions   Phlebitis and inflammation at the site of injection, pruritus, rash, fever, toxic epidermal necrolysis, Stevens–Johnson syndrome, and erythema multiforme have been reported with cephalosporin antibiotics, including ceftazidime. Angioedema and anaphylaxis (bronchospasm and/or hypotension) have been reported very rarely. Diarrhea, nausea, vomiting, abdominal pain, pseudomembranous colitis, headache, dizziness, paresthesia, seizures, encephalopathy, coma, asterixis, neuromuscular excitability, myoclonia, candidiasis, vaginitis, hemolytic anemia, hemolytic anemia, eosinophilia, thrombocytosis. Slight elevations in one or more of the hepatic enzymes. Elevations of blood urea, blood urea nitrogen, and/or serum creatinine. Transient leukopenia, neutropenia, agranulocytosis, thrombocytopenia, and lymphocytosis.

Pregnancy Category   B.
Drug Interactions   Excreted in human milk in low concentrations. Caution should be exercised when administered to a nursing woman.

Ceftriaxone

Brand Name   Rocephin.
Class of Drug   Antibiotic.
Indications   LRIs—caused by S. pneumoniae, S. aureus, H. influenzae, H. parainfluenzae, K. pneumoniae, E. coli, Enterobacter aerogenes, P. mirabilis, S. marcescens. Acute bacterial otitis media—caused by S. pneumoniae, H. influenzae (including beta-lactamase-producing strains), M. catarrhalis (including beta-lactamase-producing strains). Skin and skin structure infections—caused by S. aureus, Staphylococcus epidermidis, Streptococcus pyogenes , viridans group streptococci (VGS), E. coli, Enterobacter cloacae, Klebsiella oxytoca, Klebsiella pneumoniae, P. mirabilis, Morganella morganii*, P. aeruginosa, S. marcescens, A. calcoaceticus, B. fragilis*, Peptostreptococcus spp. UTIs (complicated and uncomplicated)—caused by E. coli, P. mirabilis, Proteus vulgaris, M. morganii, or K. pneumoniae. Uncomplicated gonorrhea (cervical/urethral and rectal)—caused by Neisseria gonorrhoeae, including both penicillinase- and non-penicillinase-producing strains Pharyngeal gonorrhea—caused by non-penicillinase-producing strains of N. gonorrhoeae. Pelvic inflammatory disease—caused by N. gonorrhoeae. Rocephin, like other cephalosporins, has no activity against Chlamydia trachomatis; therefore, when cephalosporins are used in the treatment of patients with pelvic inflammatory disease and C. trachomatis is one of the suspected pathogens, appropriate antichlamydial coverage should be added. Bacterial septicemia—caused by S. aureus, S. pneumoniae, E. coli, H. influenzae, K. pneumoniae. Bone and joint infections—caused by S. aureus, S. pneumoniae, E. coli, P. mirabilis, K. pneumoniae, Enterobacter spp. Intra-abdominal infections—caused by E. coli, K. pneumoniae, B. fragilis, Clostridium spp. (note: most strains of Clostridium difficile colitis are resistant), Peptostreptococcus spp. Meningitis—caused by H. influenzae, N. meningitidis, S. pneumoniae. Has also been used successfully in a limited number of cases of meningitis and shunt infection caused by

S. epidermidis* and *E. coli**. (*Efficacy for this organism in this organ system was studied in fewer than ten infections.)

Surgical prophylaxis—preoperative administration of a single 1-g dose may reduce the incidence of postoperative infections in patients undergoing surgical procedures classified as contaminated or potentially contaminated (e.g., vaginal or abdominal hysterectomy or cholecystectomy for chronic calculous cholecystitis in high-risk patients, such as those older than 70 years of age, with acute cholecystitis not requiring therapeutic antimicrobials, obstructive jaundice, or common bile duct stones) and in surgical patients for whom infection at the operative site would present serious risk (e.g., during coronary artery bypass surgery). Although Rocephin has been shown to have been as effective as cefazolin in the prevention of infection following coronary artery bypass surgery, no placebo-controlled trials have been conducted to evaluate any cephalosporin antibiotic in the prevention of infection following coronary artery bypass surgery.

Dosage Form Sterile solution for injection.

Dose *Adult minimum:maximum:* 0.25 g:4.0 g. *Pediatric minimum: maximum:* 0.025 g/kg:0.1 g/kg. *Adults:* The usual adult daily dose is 1–2 g given once per day (or in equally divided doses two times per day), depending on the type and severity of infection. Total daily dose should not exceed 4 g. If *C. trachomatis* is a suspected pathogen, appropriate antichlamydial coverage should be added because ceftriaxone sodium has no activity against this organism. For the treatment of uncomplicated gonococcal infections, a single i.m. dose of 250 mg is recommended. For preoperative use (surgical prophylaxis), a single dose of 1 g administered i.v. 1/2–2 h before surgery is recommended. *Pediatric:* For the treatment of skin and skin structure infections, the recommended total daily dose is 50–75 mg/kg given once per day (or in equally divided doses two times per day). The total daily dose should not exceed 2 g. For the treatment of acute bacterial otitis media, a single i.m. dose of 50 mg/kg (not to exceed 1 g) is recommended. For the treatment of serious miscellaneous infections other than meningitis, the recommended total daily dose is 50–75 mg/kg given in divided doses every 12 h. The total daily dose should not exceed 2 g. In the treatment of meningitis, it is recommended that the initial therapeutic dose be 100 mg/kg (not to exceed 4 g). Thereafter, a total daily dose of 100 mg/kg per day (not to exceed 4 g per day) is recommended. The daily dose may be administered once per day (or in equally divided doses every 12 h). The usual duration of therapy is 7–14 days. Generally, therapy should be continued for at least 2 days after the signs and symptoms of infection have disappeared. The usual duration of therapy is 4–14 days; in complicated infections, longer therapy may be required. When treating infections caused by *S. pyogenes*, therapy should be continued for at least 10 days.

Contraindications   Blood coagulation disorder, diseases of the liver, gastrointestinal disorders, malnutrition, patients with a known allergy to the cephalosporin class of antibiotics.

Warnings   Pseudomembranous colitis has been reported with nearly all antibacterial agents, including ceftriaxone, and may range in severity from mild to life threatening. Therefore, it is important to consider this diagnosis in patients who present with diarrhea subsequent to the administration of antibacterial agents.

Adverse Reactions   *Most frequent*: vulvovaginal candidiasis. *Less frequent*: abdominal pain with cramps, diarrhea, nausea, oral candidiasis, vomiting. *Rare*: allergic reactions, anaphylaxis, angioedema, choledocholithiasis, *C. difficile* colitis, drug fever, erythema, erythema multiforme, hemolytic anemia, hypoprothrombinemia, pruritus, renal disease, seizure disorder, serum sickness, skin rash, Stevens–Johnson syndrome.

Pregnancy Category   B.

Drug Interactions   Low concentrations of ceftriaxone are excreted in human milk. Caution should be exercised when administered to a nursing woman. Safety and effectiveness in neonates, infants, and pediatric patients have not been established. Should not be administered to hyperbilirubinemic neonates, especially premature infants.

Cefuroxime

Brand Name   Ceftin; Kefurox; Zinacef.

Class of Drug   Oral antibiotic. Cephalosporins.

Indications   Staphylococci, group B streptococci,*H. influenzae, E. coli, Enterobacter* spp., salmonella, and *Klebsiella* spp.; treatment of susceptible infections of lower respiratory tract, urinary tract, skin and soft tissue, bone and joint; otitis media; sepsis and gonorrhea; maxillary sinusitis in pediatric patients 3 months to 12 years of age; pharyngitis; tonsillitis; impetigo.

Dosage Form   *Injection*: 750 mg, 1.5 g. *Tablets*: (axetil) 125, 250, 500 mg.

Dose   *Children older than 3 months and up to 12 years of age*: Pharyngitis, tonsillitis—oral tablet 125 mg every 12 h for 10 days. Acute bacterial maxillary sinusitis—oral tablet 250 mg two times per day for 10 days. Acute otitis media—oral tablet 250 mg two times per day for 10 days; i.m. or i.v. 75–150 mg/kg per day divided every 8 h. *Children older than 12 years of age and adults*: oral tablet 250–500 mg two times per day for 10 days. *Early Lyme disease*: oral tablet 500 mg two times per day for 20 days; i.m. and i.v. 750 mg to 1.5 g per dose every 8 h.

Contraindications Zinacef in patients with known allergy to the cephalosporin group of antibiotics.

Warnings Increased serum levels with probenecid; aminoglycosides increase nephrotoxicity.

Adverse Reactions Thrombophlebitis, decreased hemoglobin and hematocrit, eosinophilia, increased liver enzymes (1–10% of patients); anaphylaxis, angioedema, cholestasis, colitis, diarrhea, dizziness, erythema multiforme, fever, GI bleeding, headache, hemolytic anemia, increased BUN, increased creatinine, interstitial nephritis, leucopenia, nausea, neutropenia, pain at injection site, pancytopenia, prolonged PT, pseudomembranous colitis, rash, seizures, stomach cramps, thrombocytopenia, vaginitis, vomiting (less than 1% of patients).

Pregnancy Category B.

Drug Interactions Concomitant administration of probenecid with cefuroxime axetil tablets increases the area under the serum concentration versus time curve by 50%. Drugs that reduce gastric acidity may result in a lower bioavailability of Ceftin compared with that of fasting state and tend to cancel the effect of postprandial absorption.

Chlorambucil

Brand Name Leukeran.

Class of Drug Nitrogen mustard family of alkylating agents. Inhibits T- and B-cell proliferation by causing DNA–DNA cross-linkage.

Indications Chronic lymphatic (lymphocytic) leukemia; malignant lymphomas, including lymphosarcoma, giant follicular lymphoma, Hodgkin's disease; primary (Waldenström's) macroglobulinemia. Sometimes used to treat vasculitic complications of rheumatoid arthritis, autoimmune hemolytic anemias associated with cold agglutinins. Ocular or neurological Adamantiades–Behçet disease and various other forms of uveitis that are recalcitrant to conventional therapy. May be effective in the treatment of sympathetic ophthalmia. Intractable JRA-associated iridocyclitis has shown to be responsive.

Dosage Form Tablet.

Dose 0.1–0.2 mg/kg per day. Prefer to begin with a dose of 0.1 mg/kg per day, titrating the dose based on clinical response and drug tolerance every 3 weeks for a maximum dose of 18 mg/day. Complications, such as myelosuppression, increase significantly at doses greater than 10 mg/day. Monitor CBC with differential, ALT, and AST weekly for first month (or until appropriate WBC count is achieved) then every 2–4 weeks.

Contraindications   In patients whose disease has demonstrated prior resistance to the agent. Patients who have demonstrated hypersensitivity to chlorambucil should not be given the drug. May be cross-hypersensitivity (skin rash) between chlorambucil and other alkylating agents.

Warnings   Convulsions, infertility, leukemia, and secondary malignancies have been observed when employed in the therapy of malignant and nonmalignant diseases.

Adverse Reactions   Bone marrow suppression, infection, gastrointestinal upset. *Reproductive*: Gonadal dysfunction—oligospermia, azoospermia, potentially irreversible ovarian dysfunction resulting in a medication-induced menopause, infertility. *Neurologic*: Tremors, muscular twitching, myoclonia, confusion, agitation, ataxia, flaccid paresis, hallucinations; resolve upon discontinuation. In rare instances, focal and/or generalized seizures have been reported in both children and adults. *Dermatologic*: allergic reactions, such as urticaria and angioneurotic edema, have been reported following initial or subsequent dosing; skin hypersensitivity (including rare reports of skin rash progressing to erythema multiforme, toxic epidermal necrolysis, and Stevens–Johnson syndrome) has been reported. *Miscellaneous*: pulmonary fibrosis, hepatotoxicity and jaundice, drug fever, peripheral neuropathy, interstitial pneumonia, sterile cystitis, infertility, leukemia, and secondary malignancies.

Pregnancy Category   D.

Drug Interactions   Potential teratogen and has been reported to cause urogenital abnormalities in the offspring of mothers receiving this drug during the first trimester of pregnancy. Whether the drug is excreted in the human milk is not known. No known drug–drug interactions. Safety and effectiveness in pediatric patients have not been established.

Chloramphenicol

Brand Name   Chloroptic; Chloromycetin; Ocu-chlor.

Class of Drug   Antibiotic. Inhibits bacterial protein synthesis.

Indications   Surface ocular infections involving the conjunctiva and/or cornea caused by chloramphenicol-susceptible organisms; active against *S. aureus.*; streptococci, including *S. pneumoniae*; *E. coli*; *H. influenzae*; *Klebsiella/Enterobacter* spp.; *Moraxella lacunata* (Morax-Axenfeld bacillus); *Neisseria* spp. Products do not provide adequate coverage against *P. aeruginosa* or *S. marcescens*.

Dosage Form	Topical ophthalmic solution 05%. Topical ophthalmic ointment 1%.
Dose	*Solution*: 1–2 drops every 3 h, or more frequently if deemed advisable. *Ointment*: A small amount placed in the eye every 3 h, or more frequently if deemed advisable. Administration should be continued day and night for the first 48 h, after which the interval between applications may be increased. Treatment should be continued for at least 48 h after the eye appears normal.
Contraindications	In persons sensitive to the product or any of its components.
Warnings	Bone marrow hypoplasia, including aplastic anemia and death, has been reported following local application. Should not be used when agents less-potentially dangerous would be expected to provide effective treatment.
Adverse Reactions	Blood dyscrasias have been reported (see »Warnings«).*Solution*: transient burning or stinging sensations may occur. *Ointment*: allergic or inflammatory reactions due to individual hypersensitivity and occasional burning or stinging may occur.
Pregnancy Category	C.

Cidofovir

Brand Name	Vistide.
Class of Drug	Antiviral.
Indications	Cytomegalovirus (CMV) retinitis in patients with acquired immunodeficiency syndrome (AIDS).*Safety and efficacy have not been established for treatment of other CMV infections (such as pneumonitis or gastroenteritis), congenital or neonatal CMV disease, or CMV disease in non-HIV-infected individuals.*
Dosage Form	Injection.
Dose	*Induction*: 5 mg/kg body weight (given as an i.v. infusion at a constant rate over 1 h) administered once weekly for two consecutive weeks. It is important to utilize the Cockcroft–Gault formula to more precisely estimate CrCl and the patient's underlying renal status. *Maintenance*: 5 mg/kg body weight (given as an i.v. infusion at a constant rate over 1 hr), administered once every 2 weeks. *Dose adjustment*: Changes in renal function—maintenance dose must be reduced from 5 mg/kg to 3 mg/kg for an increase in serum creatinine of 0.3–0.4 mg/dl above baseline; must be discontinued for an increase in serum creatinine of ≥0.5 mg/dl above baseline or development of ≥3+ proteinuria. *Probenecid*: must be administered orally with each dose; 2 g must be administered 3 h prior to the Vistide dose and 1 g administered at 2 h and again at 8 h after completion of the 1-h infusion (for a total of 4 g).

Hydration: Patients must receive at least 1 l of 0.9% (normal) saline solution i.v. with each infusion of Vistide. The saline solution should be infused over a 1- to 2-h period immediately before Vistide infusion. Patients who can tolerate the additional fluid load should receive a second liter; if administered, the second liter should be initiated either at the start of the Vistide infusion or immediately afterward and infused over a 1- to 3-h period. *Patient monitoring*: Serum creatinine and urine protein must be monitored within 48 h prior to each dose. WBCs with differential should be monitored prior to each dose. In patients with proteinuria, i.v. hydration should be administered and the test repeated. IOP, visual acuity, and ocular symptoms should be monitored periodically.

Contraindications
Direct intraocular injection: direct injection of cidofovir has been associated with iritis, ocular hypotony, and permanent impairment of vision. Initiation of therapy with Vistide is contraindicated in patients with a serum creatinine >1.5 mg/dl, a calculated CrCl ≤55 ml/min, or a urine protein ≥100 mg/dl (equivalent to ≥2+ proteinuria); in patients receiving agents with nephrotoxic potential (such agents must be discontinued at least 7 days prior to starting therapy); in patients with hypersensitivity to cidofovir; in patients with a history of clinically severe hypersensitivity to probenecid or other sulfa-containing medications.

Warnings
Nephrotoxicity: Cases of acute renal failure resulting in dialysis and/or contributing to death have occurred with as few as one or two doses of Vistide. Renal function (serum creatinine and urine protein) must be monitored within 48 h prior to each dose. Dose adjustment or discontinuation is required for changes in renal function. Proteinuria, as measured by urinalysis in a clinical laboratory, may be an early indicator of Vistide-related nephrotoxicity. IV normal saline hydration and oral probenecid must accompany each Vistide infusion. Doses greater than the recommended dose must not be administered, and the frequency or rate of administration must not be exceeded. *Hematological toxicity*: neutropenia may occur, and neutrophil count should be monitored during therapy. *Decreased IOP/ocular hypotony*: Decreased IOP may occur and in some instances has been associated with decreased visual acuity. IOP should be monitored during therapy. *Metabolic acidosis*: Decreased serum bicarbonate associated with proximal tubule injury and renal wasting syndrome (including Fanconi's syndrome) have been reported. Cases of metabolic acidosis in association with liver dysfunction and pancreatitis resulting in death have been reported. Uveitis or iritis was reported in clinical trials and during postmarketing. Treatment with topical corticosteroids with or without topical cycloplegic agents should be considered.

Adverse Reactions
Ocular: Decreased IOP/ocular hypotony—Among the subset of patients monitored for IOP changes, a ≥50% decrease from

baseline was reported in 17 of 70 (24%) patients at the 5 mg/ kg maintenance dose. Severe hypotony (IOP of 0–1 mmHg) was reported in three patients. Risk of ocular hypotony may be increased in patients with preexisting diabetes mellitus. Anterior uveitis/iritis—Has been reported in clinical trials and during postmarketing; reported in 15 of 135 (11%) patients receiving 5 mg/kg maintenance dosing. Treatment with topical corticosteroids with or without topical cycloplegic agents may be considered. Patients should be monitored for signs and symptoms of uveitis/iritis. *Nonocular*: Other systemic adverse reactions—fever, infection, pneumonia, dyspnea, nausea, vomiting, nephrotoxicity, neutropenia, Fanconi's syndrome, proteinuria, metabolic acidosis. Cases of metabolic acidosis in association with liver dysfunction and pancreatitis resulting in death have been reported.

Pregnancy Category C.

Drug Interactions Other drugs toxic to the kidneys should not be taken concomitantly.

Ciprofloxacin Hydrochloride

Brand Name Ciloxan.

Class of Drug Antibiotic. Interferes with DNA gyrase.

Indications *Solution*: Corneal ulcers—caused by *P. aeruginosa*, *S. marcescens**, *S. aureus*, *S. epidermidis*, *S. pneumoniae*, VGS*. Conjunctivitis—caused by *H. influenzae*, *S. aureus*, *S. epidermidis*, *S. pneumoniae*. *Ointment*: bacterial conjunctivitis caused by susceptible strains of the following microorganisms: Grampositive—*S. aureus*, *S. epidermidis*, *S. pneumoniae*, VSG; gramnegative—*H. influenzae*. (*Efficacy for this organism was studied in fewer than ten infections.)

Dosage Form Topical ophthalmic solution 0.3%. Topical ophthalmic ointment 0.3%.

Dose *Solution*: Corneal ulcers—2 drops to affected eye every 15 min for the first 6 h and then 2 drops every 30 min for the remainder of the first day. On the second day, 2 drops to affected eye hourly. On the third through 14th day, 2 drops to affected eye every 4 h. Treatment may be continued after 14 days if corneal re-epithelialization has not occurred. Bacterial conjunctivitis—1–2 drops every 2 h while awake for 2 days, and 1 or 2 drops every 4 h while awake for the next 5 days. *Ointment*: 1-cm (approx. ½-in.) ribbon three times per day to the affected eye(s) on the first 2 days, then apply a 1-cm (approx. ½-in.). ribbon two times per day for the next 5 days.

Contraindications	In persons with a history of hypersensitivity to the product or any of its components or to any member of the quinolone class of antimicrobial agents.
Warnings	Serious and occasionally fatal hypersensitivity (anaphylactic) reactions, some following the first dose, have been reported in patients receiving systemic quinolone therapy. Some reactions were accompanied by cardiovascular collapse, loss of consciousness, tingling, pharyngeal or facial edema, dyspnea, urticaria, and itching. Only a few patients had a history of hypersensitivity reactions. Serious anaphylactic reactions require immediate emergency treatment with epinephrine and other resuscitation measures, including oxygen, i.v. fluids, i.v. antihistamines, corticosteroids, pressor amines, and airway management, as clinically indicated. Remove contact lenses before using.
Adverse Reactions	*Ocular*: Most frequent—local burning or discomfort. In corneal ulcer studies with frequent administration of the drug, white crystalline precipitates were seen in approximately 17% of patients. Other reactions—lid-margin crusting, crystals/scales, foreign-body sensation, itching, conjunctival hyperemia, and a bad taste (less than 10% of patients); additional events occurring in less than 1% of patients included corneal staining, keratopathy/keratitis, allergic reactions, lid edema, tearing, photophobia, corneal infiltrates, nausea, and decreased vision. In manufacturer trials, in patients with corneal ulcers, a white crystalline precipitate located in the superficial portion of the corneal defect was observed in 35 (16.6%) of 210 patients. The onset of the precipitate was within 24 h to 7 days after starting therapy. In 17 patients, resolution of the precipitate was seen in 1–8 days. In five patients, resolution was noted in 10–13 days. In nine patients, exact resolution days were unavailable; however, at follow-up examinations 18–44 days after onset of the event, complete resolution of the precipitate was noted. In three patients, outcome information was unavailable. The precipitate did not preclude continued use of ciprofloxacin nor did it adversely affect the clinical course of the ulcer or visual outcome. *Systemic*: occurred at an incidence below 1% and included dermatitis, nausea, and taste perversion.
Pregnancy Category	C.
Drug Interactions	Long-term carcinogenicity studies in mice and rats have been completed. After daily oral dosing for up to 2 years, there was no evidence of any carcinogenic or tumorigenic effects in these species. Specific drug interaction studies have not been conducted with ophthalmic ciprofloxacin. However, systemic administration of some quinolones has been shown to elevate plasma concentrations of theophylline, interfere with the metabolism of caffeine, enhance the effects of the oral anticoagulant warfarin and its derivatives, and has been

associated with transient elevations in serum creatinine in patients receiving cyclosporine concomitantly.

Clindamycin

Brand Name	Cleocin; Pediatric.
Class of Drug	Antibiotic.
Indications	*Anaerobes*: serious respiratory tract infections (RTIs), such as empyema, anaerobic pneumonitis, and lung abscess; serious skin and soft tissue infections; septicemia; intra-abdominal infections, such as peritonitis and intra-abdominal abscess (typically resulting from anaerobic organisms resident in the normal gastrointestinal tract); infections of the female pelvis and genital tract, such as endometritis, nongonococcal tuboovarian abscess, pelvic cellulitis, and postsurgical vaginal-cuff infection. *Streptococci*: serious RTIs, serious skin and soft tissue infections. *Staphylococci*: serious RTIs, serious skin and soft tissue infections. *Pneumococci*: serious RTIs.
Dosage Form	See section on Oral Antibiotics (e.g., Cefuroxime).
Dose	*Adults*: Serious infections—150–300 mg every 6 h. More severe infections—300–450 mg every 6 h. *Pediatric patients*: Serious infections—8–16 mg/kg per day (4–8 mg/lb per day) divided into three or four equal doses. More severe infections—16–20 mg/kg per day (8–10 mg/lb per day) divided into three or four equal doses.
Contraindications	In patients with a history of hypersensitivity to preparations containing clindamycin or lincomycin. *Most significant*: Crohn's disease, *C. difficile* colitis, ulcerative colitis. *Significant*: severe hepatic disease. *Possibly significant*: atopic dermatitis, diarrhea, severe renal disease.
Warnings	Because therapy has been associated with severe colitis that may end fatally, it should be reserved for serious infections where less toxic antimicrobial agents are inappropriate. It should not be used in patients with nonbacterial infections, such as most URTIs.
Adverse Reactions	*Gastrointestinal*: abdominal pain, pseudomembranous colitis, esophagitis, nausea, vomiting, and diarrhea. *Hypersensitivity reactions*: Generalized mild to moderate morbilliform-like (maculopapular) skin rashes are the most frequently reported. Vesiculobullous rashes, as well as urticaria, have been observed. Rare instances of erythema multiforme, some resembling Stevens–Johnson syndrome, and a few cases of anaphylactoid reactions have also been reported. *Skin and mucous membranes*: pruritus, vaginitis, and rare instances of exfoliative dermatitis have been reported. *Liver*: jaundice and

abnormalities in LFTs have been observed. *Renal*: although no direct relationship to renal damage has been established, renal dysfunction as evidenced by azotemia, oliguria, and/or proteinuria has been observed in rare instances. *Hematopoietic*: Transient neutropenia (leukopenia) and eosinophilia have been reported. Reports of agranulocytosis and thrombocytopenia have been made. No direct etiologic relationship to concurrent clindamycin therapy could be made in any of the foregoing. *Musculoskeletal*: rare instances of polyarthritis have been reported.

Pregnancy Category B.

Drug Interactions Reported to appear in human milk in the range of 0.7–3.8 mcg/ml. When administered to the pediatric population (birth to 16 years of age), appropriate monitoring of organ system functions is desirable.

Cocaine

Brand Name Cocaine Hydrochloride.

Class of Drug Topical local anesthetic. Blocks norepinephrine reuptake.

Indications Local anesthetic (not for ocular use). Diagnostic testing of Horner's syndrome (2–10%).

Dosage Form Aqueous solution.

Dose Each milliliter contains cocaine hydrochloride 40 mg or 100 mg.

Contraindications In patients with a known history of hypersensitivity to the product or to any of its components or patients with compromised cardiovascular or cerebrovascular status.

Warnings *Resuscitative equipment and drugs should be immediately available when any local anesthetic is used.*

Adverse Reactions May be due to high plasma levels as a result of excessive and rapid absorption. Reactions are systemic in nature and involve the CNS and/or the cardiovascular system. A small number of reactions may result from hypersensitivity, idiosyncrasy, or diminished tolerance on the part of the patient. CNS reactions are excitatory and/or depressant and may be characterized by nervousness, restlessness, and excitement. Tremors and eventually clonic–tonic convulsions may result. Emesis may occur. Central stimulation is followed by depression, with death resulting from respiratory failure. Small doses of cocaine slow the heart rate, but after moderate doses, the rate is increased due to central sympathetic stimulation. Cocaine is pyrogenic, augmenting heat production in stimulating muscular activity and causing vasoconstriction, which decreases heat loss. Cocaine is known to interfere with the uptake of norepinephrine by adrenergic nerve terminals producing sensitization to catecholamines, causing vasoconstriction and mydriasis. Cocaine causes sloughing of the corneal epithelium, causing clouding, pitting, and occasionally ulceration of the cornea. The drug is not meant for ophthalmic use.

Pregnancy Category C.

Drug Interactions When mixed with other stimulants, including some over-the-counter cold medications, this drug can dangerously raise blood pressure. There is a danger in taking cocaine with any drug that is intended to affect heart rhythm or with drugs that raise sensitive to seizures (high doses of caffeine). This combination may cause heart attack. MAOIs increase the drug's effect, making overdose more likely.

Colchicine

Brand Name Colchicine.

Class of Drug Plant alkaloid. Inhibits neutrophil chemotaxis by inhibiting microtubule polymerization.

Indications Gout. Drug of choice for familial Mediterranean fever. Effective in a variety of dermatologic and systemic diseases, such as psoriasis, Adamantiades–Behçet disease, prophylaxis of recurrent ocular and systemic manifestations of Adamantiades–Behçet disease.

Dosage Form *Oral tablets*: 0.5 mg, 0.6 mg. *Sterile solution for i.v. injection*: 0.5 mg/ml.

Dose 1–2 mg/day or 0.5–0.6 mg orally two to three times/day.

Contraindications In patients who have serious gastrointestinal, renal, hepatic, or cardiac disorders, especially in the presence of combined kidney and liver disease. Administer with great caution in the elderly. In patients with hypersensitivity reaction to the drug. Should not be used during pregnancy and used with caution when administered to nursing mothers.

Warnings Has a very narrow therapeutic window. Can cause fetal harm when administered to a pregnant woman: if used during pregnancy, or if the patient becomes pregnant while taking it, the woman should be apprised of the potential hazard to the fetus.*Mortality related to overdosage*: cumulative i.v. doses above 4 mg have resulted in irreversible multiple organ failure and death.

Adverse Reactions Side effects are dose dependent. Gastrointestinal disturbances may lead to electrolyte imbalance (nausea/vomiting, abdominal cramping, hyperperistalsis, watery diarrhea). Alopecia, agranulocytosis (rare), leukopenia, aplastic anemia, thrombocytopenia, muscular weakness, myopathy, peripheral neuritis, urticaria, purpura alopecia. azoospermia, megal-oblastic anemia secondary to vitamin B_{12} malabsorption. Overdose can cause irreversible multiorgan failure and death, and there is usually a latent period between overdosage and the onset of symptoms. Monitor CBC with differential, ALT, and AST every 2 weeks for the first month then every 4–6 weeks.

Pregnancy Category D.

Drug Interactions Safety and effectiveness in children have not been establis-hed. Has been shown to induce reversible malabsorption of vitamin B_{12}, apparently by altering the function of ileal mu-cosa. The possibility that colchicine may increase response to CNS depressants and to sympathomimetic agents is sugges-ted by the results of experiments on animals. Should not be used during pregnancy and used with caution when admi-nistered to nursing mothers.

Colistimethate Sodium

Brand Name Coly-Mycin M Parenteral.

Class of Drug Antibiotic.

Indications Treatment of acute or chronic infections due to sensitive strains of certain gram-negative bacilli. It is particularly indi-cated when the infection is caused by sensitive strains of *P. aeruginosa*. This antibiotic is not indicated for infections due to *Proteus* or *Neisseria*. Proven clinically effective in treatment of infections due to the following gram-negative organisms: *E. aerogenes, E. coli, K. pneumoniae* , and *P. aeruginosa*. May be used to initiate therapy in serious infections suspected to be due to gram-negative organisms and in the treatment of infections due to susceptible gram-negative pathogenic ba-cilli.

Dose Maximum daily dose should not exceed 5 mg/kg (2.3 mg/lb) with normal renal function.*Adults and pediatric patients*: i.v. or i.m. *Administration*: should be given in 2–4 divided doses at dose levels of 2.5–5 mg/kg per day for patients with normal renal function, depending on the severity of the infection. In obese individuals, dosage should be based on ideal body weight. Daily dose should be reduced in the presence of renal impairment.

Contraindications In patients with a history of sensitivity to the product or any of its components.

Warnings Overdosage can result in renal insufficiency, muscle weak-ness, and apnea. Respiratory arrest has been reported follo-wing i.m. administration of colistimethate sodium. Impaired renal function increases the possibility of apnea and neuro-muscular blockade following administration.

Adverse Reactions   *Gastrointestinal*: gastrointestinal upset. *Nervous system*: ting-ling of extremities and tongue, slurred speech, dizziness, vertigo, paresthesia. *Integumentary*: generalized itching, ur-ticaria, rash. *Body as a whole*: fever. *Laboratory deviations*: in-creased BUN, elevated creatinine, decreased CrCl. *Respiratory system*: respiratory distress, apnea. *Renal system*: nephrotoxi-city, decreased urine output.

Pregnancy Category   C.

Drug Interactions   It is not known whether this drug is excreted in human milk. However, colistin sulfate is excreted in human milk. Therefore, caution should be exercised when colistimethate sodium is administered to nursing women. In clinical studies, colistime-thate sodium was administered to the pediatric population (neonates, infants, children, adolescents). Although adverse reactions appear to be similar in the adult and pediatric po-pulations, subjective symptoms of toxicity may not be repor-ted by pediatric patients. Close clinical monitoring of pedia-tric patients is recommended.

Corticosteroids

Class of Drug   Anti-inflammatory. Immunosuppressant. Cytoplasmic stero-id receptor complexes bind to DNA glucocorticoid response elements (GREs) and control the transcription of specific ge-nes.

Indications   Uveitis.

Dosage Form   *Oral*: prednisone. *IV*: methylprednisone dexamethasone.

Dose   *Oral*: prednisone 0.5–1.5 mg/kg per day tapered over weeks to months as inflammation is controlled, or add steroid-spa-ring agent if more than10–20 mg/day is needed to control inflammation. *IV*: megadose for severe life-threatening or vi-sion-threatening uveitis, methylprednisolone 250–1,000 mg/day for up to 3 days.

Contraindications

Warnings   Avoid prolonged use, especially in children, in whom growth retardation can occur quite rapidly.

Adverse Reactions   Adrenal suppression and insufficiency, altered mood or men-tation, systemic hypertension, elevated blood sugars, hypo-kalemia, leukocytosis, weight gain, myopathy, osteoporosis. Monitor blood pressure, serum electrolytes, fasting glucose level; monitoring and preventive measures for osteoporosis.

Pregnancy Category   B.

Cromolyn Sodium

Brand Name	Crolom; Opticrom.
Class of Drug	Mast-cell stabilizer.
Indications	Vernal keratoconjunctivitis, vernal conjunctivitis, vernal keratitis.
Dosage Form	Topical ophthalmic solution 4%.
Dose	1–2 drops in each eye four to six times per day at regular intervals.
Contraindications	In patients who have shown hypersensitivity to the product or to any of its components.
Adverse Reactions	Most frequently reported attributed to the use of cromolyn sodium ophthalmic solution, on the basis of reoccurrence following readministration, is transient ocular stinging or burning upon instillation. Reported as infrequent events; it is unclear whether they are attributed to the drug: conjunctival injection, watery eyes, itchy eyes, dryness around the eye, puffy eyes, eye irritation, and styes. Immediate hypersensitivity reactions have been reported rarely and include dyspnea, edema, and rash.
Pregnancy Category	B.
Drug Interactions	In animals receiving parenteral cromolyn, adverse fetal effects were noted only at very high parenteral doses, which produced maternal toxicity. It is not known whether this drug is excreted in human milk. Because many drugs are excreted in human milk, caution should be exercised when administering to a nursing woman. Safety and effectiveness in pediatric patients younger than 4 years of age have not been established.

Cyclopentolate Hydrochloride

Brand Name	AK-Pentolate; Cyclogyl; Cylate.
Class of Drug	Cycloplegic/mydriatic. Anticholinergic.
Indications	Cycloplegic refraction, anterior uveitis, postoperative cycloplegia, fundus examination.
Dosage Form	Topical ophthalmic solution 0.5%, 1%, 2%.
Dose	*Adults*: 1–2 drops of 0.5%, 1%, or 2% concentration, which may be repeated in 5–10 min, if necessary; complete recovery usually occurs in 24 h. *Children*: 1–2 drops of 0.5%, 1%, or 2% concentration, which may be repeated 5–10 min later, if necessary. *Small infants*: single instillation of 1 drop of 0.5%

concentration; to minimize absorption, apply pressure over the nasolacrimal sac for 2–3 min and observe infant closely for at least 30 min. Individuals with heavily pigmented irides may require higher strengths.

Contraindications   Should not be used when narrow-angle glaucoma (NAG) or anatomical narrow angles are present or where there is hypersensitivity to the product or any of its components.

Warnings   May cause CNS disturbances. This is especially true in younger age groups but may occur at any age, especially with stronger solutions. Premature and small infants are especially prone to CNS and cardiopulmonary side effects from systemic absorption. To minimize absorption, use only 1 drop of 0.5% concentration per eye followed by pressure applied over the nasolacrimal sac for 2–3 min; observe infants closely for at least 30 min. Patient should be advised not to drive or engage in other hazardous activities while pupils are dilated.

Adverse Reactions   *Ocular*: increased IOP, burning, photophobia, blurred vision, irritation, hyperemia, conjunctivitis, blepharoconjunctivitis, punctate keratitis, synechiae. *Systemic*: Has been associated with psychotic reactions and behavioral disturbances, usually in children, especially with 2% concentration. These disturbances include ataxia, incoherent speech, restlessness, hallucinations, hyperactivity, seizures, disorientation as to time and place, and failure to recognize people. Produces reactions similar to those of other anticholinergic drugs, but the CNS manifestations as noted above are more common. *Other toxic manifestations* of anticholinergic drugs are skin rash, abdominal discretion in infants, unusual drowsiness, tachycardia, hyperpyrexia, vasodilation, urinary retention, diminished gastrointestinal motility, and decreased secretion in salivary and sweat glands, pharynx, bronchi, and nasal passages. *Severe manifestations* of toxicity include coma, medullary paralysis, and death.

Pregnancy Category   C.

Drug Interactions   May interfere with the antiglaucoma action of carbachol or pilocarpine; also, concurrent use of these medications may antagonize the antiglaucoma and miotic actions of ophthalmic cholinesterase inhibitors. Increased susceptibility to cyclopentolate has been reported in infants, young children, and children with spastic paralysis or brain damage. Therefore, cyclopentolate should be used with great caution in these patients. Feeding intolerance may follow ophthalmic use of this product in neonates. It is recommended that feeding be withheld for 4 h after examination. Do not use in concentrations higher than 0.5% in small infants.

Brand Name   Cyclomydril (cyclopentolate HCl, phenylephrine HCl).

Class of Drug   Cycloplegic/mydriatic. Anticholinergic, alpha-adrenergic agonist.

Indications   For the production of mydriasis.

Dosage Form   Topical ophthalmic solution. Cyclopentolate 0.2%, phenyle-
                         phrine 1%.
Dose   1 drop in each eye every 5–10 min not to exceed three times.
                         Observe infants closely for at least 30 min.
Contraindications   Do not use in patients with NAG or anatomically narrow ang-
                         les or where there is hypersensitivity to the product or any of
                         its components.
Warnings   For topical use only. The use of this combination may have
                         an adverse effect on individuals suffering from cardiovascular
                         disease, hypertension, and hyperthyroidism; and it may cause
                         CNS disturbances. Small infants are especially prone to CNS
                         and cardiopulmonary side effects from systemic absorption
                         of cyclopentolate. Patients should be advised not to drive or
                         engage in other hazardous activities while pupils are dilated.
                         Feeding intolerance may follow ophthalmic use in neonates.
                         It is recommended that feeding be withheld for 4 h after exa-
                         mination.
Adverse Reactions   See »AK-Pentolate; Cyclogyl; Cylate.« In case of severe ma-
                         nifestations of toxicity, the antidote of choice is physostig-
                         mine salicylate:*Pediatric dose*—as an antidote, slowly inject
                         i.v. 0.5 mg of physostigmine salicylate; if toxic symptoms
                         persist and no cholinergic symptoms are produced, repeat
                         at 5-min intervals to a maximum dose of 2.0 mg. *Adolescent
                         and adult dose*—as an antidote, slowly inject i.v. 2.0 mg of
                         physostigmine salicylate; a second dose of 1–2 mg may be
                         given after 20 min if no reversal of toxic manifestations has
                         occurred.
Pregnancy Category   C.

Cyclophosphamide

Brand Name   Cytoxan; Neosar.
Class of Drug   Nitrogen mustard family of alkylating agents. Inhibits T- and
                         B-cell proliferation by causing DNA–DNA cross linkage.
Indications   Cancer of breast and ovary; lymphoma; leukemia; multiple
                         myeloma; mycosis fungoides; nephrotic syndrome; neu-
                         roblastoma; retinoblastoma; Wegener's granulomatosis;
                         polyarteritis nodosa; highly destructive forms of ocular in-
                         flammation (peripheral ulcerative keratitis) associated with
                         rheumatoid arthritis; necrotizing scleritis; peripheral keratitis;
                         bilateral Mooren's ulcer; patients with active, progressive,
                         ocular cicatricial pemphigoid (OCP); Adamantiades–Behçet
                         disease with posterior uveitis or retinal vasculitis manifesta-
                         tions; pars planitis.
Dosage Form   Oral and injectable.

Dose

1–3 mg/kg per day (dose usually titrated to target WBC of 3,000–4,000).*Ocular disease*: p.o.—1–2 mg/kg per day; i.v.—1 g/m^2 body surface area in 250 ml normal saline piggy-backed onto the second half of 1 l 0.5% dextrose in water infused in a 2-h period. Repeat every 3–4 weeks, depending on the clinical response and the nadir of the leukocyte count. Monitor urinalysis, CBC with differential, ALT, and AST weekly for first month (or until appropriate WBC count is achieved) then every 2–4 weeks. Stop Cytoxan if hematuria occurs.

Contraindications

Continued use in patients with severely depressed bone marrow function; patients with focal chorioretinitis, herpes simplex, herpes zoster, CMV, AIDS retinopathy, toxoplasmosis, tuberculosis, fungal infections, and patients who have demonstrated a previous hypersensitivity to the product or any of its components.

Warnings

Patients should drink 2–4 l of water per day to increase urine flow and minimize toxicity. Second malignancies have developed in some patients treated with cyclophosphamide used alone or in association with other antineoplastic drugs and/ or modalities. Most frequently, they have been urinary bladder, myeloproliferative, or lymphoproliferative malignancies. Second malignancies most frequently were detected in patients treated for primary myeloproliferative or lymphoproliferative malignancies or nonmalignant disease in which immune processes are believed to be involved pathologically. In JRA-associated iridocyclitis that is unresponsive to steroids and other conventional treatments, potential risks of delayed malignancy or sterility associated with use must be considered. Because cyclophosphamide is a teratogen causing CNS and skeletal abnormalities in the fetus, contraception is advisable. Nursing mothers should be cautioned that the drug is excreted in the human milk and may exert toxic effects in their infants.

Adverse Reactions

Most common: bone marrow suppression; significant leucopenia is associated with increased risk of infection and sepsis; sterile hemorrhagic cystitis; gonadal dysfunction, including azoospermia and amenorrhea; nausea, vomiting, anorexia, and stomatitis are dose related; reversible alopecia; infections; infertility. *Less common*: include cardiac myopathy, hepatic fibrosis, impaired renal clearance of water with resultant hyponatremia, and anaphylaxis. *Ocular*: include dry eyes, blurred vision, and increased IOP.

Pregnancy Category

D.

Drug Interactions

Cyclophosphamide treatment, which causes a marked and persistent inhibition of cholinesterase activity, potentiates the effect of succinylcholine chloride. Effects of agents such as halothane, nitrous oxide, and succinylcholine are enhanced by cyclophosphamide. If a patient has been treated with cyclophosphamide within 10 days of general anesthesia, the anesthesiologist should be alerted. Cyclophosphamide is affected by drugs that induce (phenobarbital) or inhibit (allopurinol) the hepatic microsomal mixed-function oxidase system. Concurrent administration of allopurinol prolongs the serum $t^{1/2}$ of cyclophosphamide, and high doses of phenobarbital increase its metabolism and leukopenic activity. Chloramphenicol and corticosteroids may inhibit microsomal enzyme metabolism, thus blunting its action. Cyclophosphamide increases the myocardial toxicity of doxorubicin.

Cyclosporine A

Brand Name	Neoral; Sandimmune; Sandoz.
Class of Drug	Immunosuppressant.
Indications	*Ocular immune-medicated disorders*: bilateral, sight-threatening uveitis of the noninfectious etiology when both the retina and choroid are involved; intractable uveitis of various etiologies (including Adamantiades–Behçet disease, birdshot retinochoroidopathy, sarcoidosis, pars planitis, VKH, multiple sclerosis, sympathetic ophthalmia, idiopathic vitreitis) refractory to corticosteroid and cytotoxic agents; corneal ulceration with or without scleral melting; peripheral ulcerative keratitis associated with Wegener's granulomatosis; preventing corneal transplant rejection in high-risk eyes. *Oculocutaneous disorders* (Sjögren's syndrome and atopic keratoconjunctivitis): keratoconjunctivitis sicca.
Dosage Form	*Neoral and Sandimmune Soft Gelatin Capsules (cyclosporine capsules)*: 25 mg and 100 mg. *Neoral and Sandimmune Oral Solution (cyclosporine oral solution)*: 100 mg/ml. *Sandimmune injection (cyclosporine injection) for intravenous infusion*: 50 mg/ml.
Dose	*Oral* (capsule or oral solution): 2–5 mg/kg per day with dosage increments of 50 mg to a maximum of 5 mg/kg per day and titrate to clinical response; occasionally increase dosage to 7.5 mg/kg per day for no more than 4 weeks and taper to 5 mg/kg per day once inflammation has been controlled. *IV*: Administered at one third the oral dose.
Contraindications	In patients with hypersensitivity to the product or any of its components, uncontrolled systemic hypertension, hepatic disease, renal insufficiency, or pregnancy.
Warnings	Sandimmune and Neoral are not bioequivalent and cannot be used interchangeably without physician supervision. Sandimmune soft gelatin capsules and Sandimmune oral solution have decreased bioavailability in comparison with Neoral soft gelatin capsules. Absorption of CsA during chronic administration of Sandimmune soft gelatin capsules and

oral solution was found to be erratic. It is recommended that patients taking the soft gelatin capsules or oral solution over a period of time be monitored at repeated intervals for CsA blood levels and subsequent dose adjustments be made in order to avoid toxicity due to high levels, and possible organ rejection due to low absorption, of CsA. Unlikely to be a human teratogen but known to cross the placenta and cause growth retardation; use in pregnancy only when the potential benefit justifies risk to the fetus; avoid in nursing mothers.

Adverse Reactions   Nephrotoxicity and hypertension are the most common and worrisome side effects.*Nephrotoxicity*: increased serum creatinine with disproportionate increase in BUN, preserved urine output and sodium reabsorption, decreased CrCl. *Systemic hypertension*: Promptly responds to dosage reduction. The dose should be decreased by 25–50% if hypertension occurs. If hypertension persists, the dose should be further reduced or blood pressure should be controlled with antihypertensive agents. In most cases, blood pressure has returned to baseline when cyclosporine was discontinued. *Hematologic*: normochromic, normocytic anemia and increased sedimentation rate. *LFTs*: mild, dose-dependent increase in serum transaminases and bilirubin levels. *Others*: hyperuricemia and gouty arthritis are common among transplant recipients; increases in total serum cholesterol due to an increased low-density lipoprotein (LDL) fraction in patients treated with CsA; lymphoproliferative disease due to immunosuppression in general; increased serum prolactin levels causing gynecomastia in men and growth of benign breast adenomas in women; paresthesia and temperature hypersensitivity; nausea and vomiting; headache; hirsutism; gingival hyperplasia; neurotoxicity; reversible myopathy; increased risk of opportunistic infections with herpesviruses, *Candida*, and *Pneumocystis*. *Ocular*: decreased vision, lid erythema, nonspecific conjunctivitis, visual hallucinations, conjunctival and retinal hemorrhage.

Pregnancy Category   C.

Drug Interactions   No evidence of teratogenicity was observed in rats or rabbits receiving oral doses of CsA up to 300 mg/kg per day during organogenesis. Although no adequate and well-controlled studies have been conducted in children, patients as young as 6 months of age have received the drug with no unusual adverse effects.*Drugs that may potentiate renal dysfunction of CsA*: Antibiotics—aminoglycosides, gentamicin, tobramycin, vancomycin, ciprofloxacin, trimethoprim with sulfamethoxazole. Antineoplastics—melphalan. Antifungals—amphotericin B, ketoconazole. Anti-inflammatory drugs—NSAID, azapropazone, diclofenac, naproxen, sulindac, colchicine. Gastrointestinal agents—cimetidine, ranitidine. Immunosuppressives—tacrolimus. *Drugs that alter CsA concentrations*: Compounds that decrease cyclosporine absorption, such as orlistat should be avoided. CsA is extensively metabolized cytochrome P-450; monitoring of circulating CsA concentrations and appropriate dosage adjustment are essential when drugs that affect the activity of cytochrome P-450 and CsA are used concomitantly. *Drugs that increase CSA concentrations*: Calcium-channel blockers—diltiazem, nicardipine, verapamil. Antifungals—fluconazole, itraconazole, ketoconazole. Antibiotics—clarithromycin, erythromycin, quinupristin/dalfopristin. Glucocorticoids—methylprednisolone. Other drugs—allopurinol, bromocriptine, danazol, metoclopramide, colchicine, amiodarone. *Drugs/dietary supplements that decrease CsA concentrations*: Antibiotics—nafcillin, rifampin. Anticonvulsants—carbamazepine, phenobarbital, phenytoin. Other drugs—octreotide, ticlopidine, orlistat, St. John's wort.

There have been reports of a serious drug interaction between CsA and the herbal dietary supplement St. John's wort, with a marked reduction in blood concentrations of CsA. Rifabutin is known to increase the metabolism of other drugs metabolized by the cytochrome P-450 system. Care should be exercised when these two drugs are administered concomitantly. Clinical status and serum creatinine should be closely monitored when CsA is used with NSAIDs in rheumatoid arthritis patients. Additive decreases in renal function have been reported. Concomitant administration of diclofenac has been associated with approximate doubling of diclofenac blood levels and occasional reports of reversible decreases in renal function. Consequently, the dose of diclofenac should be in the lower end of the therapeutic range.

Other drug interactions: Reduced clearance of prednisolone, digoxin, and lovastatin. Severe digitalis toxicity has been seen within days of starting CsA in several patients taking digoxin. CsA should not be used with potassium-sparing diuretics because hyperkalemia can occur. During treatment with CsA, vaccination may be less effective. The use of live vaccines should be avoided. Myopathy with rhabdomyolysis has occurred with concomitant lovastatin and CsA. Frequent gingival hyperplasia with nifedipine and CsA. Convulsions with high-dose methylprednisolone and CsA. Psoriasis patients receiving other immunosuppressive agents or radiation therapy, including psoralen/ultraviolet light A (PUVA) and ultraviolet light B (UVB) should not receive concurrent CsA because of the possibility of excessive immunosuppression.

Brand Name	Restasis (topical).
Class of Drug	Immunosuppressant.
Indications	Dry-eye presumed to be secondary to inflammation associated with keratoconjunctivitis sicca. Increased tear production was not seen in patients currently taking topical anti-inflammatory drugs or using punctal plugs.

Dosage Form   Cyclosporine ophthalmic emulsion 0.05%. Sterile, preservati-
                          ve free.
Dose   Invert the unit dose vial a few times to obtain a uniform,
                          white, opaque emulsion before using. Instill 1 drop two times
                          per day in each eye approximately 12 h apart. Can be used
                          concomitantly with artificial tears, allowing a 15-min interval
                          between products. Discard vial immediately after use.
Contraindications   In patients with active ocular infections and with a known or
                          suspected hypersensitivity to the product or any of its com-
                          ponents.
Warnings   Has not been studied in patients with a history of herpes ke-
                          ratitis.
Adverse Reactions   *Most common*: ocular burning (17%). *Others*: reported in
                          1–5% of patients include conjunctival hyperemia, discharge,
                          epiphora, eye pain, foreign-body sensation, pruritus, stinging,
                          and visual disturbance (most often blurring).
Pregnancy Category   Category C.
Drug Interactions   No evidence of teratogenicity was observed in rats or rabbits
                          receiving oral doses of CsA up to 300 mg/kg per day during
                          organogenesis. At doses that are 30,000–100,000 times grea-
                          ter than daily human topical Restasis doses, òral CsA induced
                          embryo- and fetotoxic effects. Systemic carcinogenicity stu-
                          dies of oral CsA in mice and rats showed increased incidence
                          of hepatocellular cancer, pancreatic adenomas, and lympho-
                          cytic cancers. CsA has not been found mutagenic/genotoxic
                          in animal studies. Safety and efficacy have not been establis-
                          hed in children younger than 16 years of age.

Daclizumab

Brand Name	Zenapax.
Class of Drug	IL-2 receptor antagonist. Binds with high-affinity to the Tac subunit of the high-affinity IL-2 receptor complex and inhibits IL-2 binding. Inhibits IL-2-mediated activation of lymphocytes.
Indications	Prophylaxis of acute organ rejection in patients receiving renal transplants. Used as part of an immunosuppressive regimen that includes cyclosporine and corticosteroids. *Off-label*: chronic, sight-threatening, refractory uveitis.
Dosage Form	Solution for i.v. injection 5 mg/ml (25 mg/5 ml).
Dose	Standard course of therapy is five doses: the first dose should be given no more than 24 h before transplantation; the four remaining doses should be given at intervals of 14 days. No dosage adjustment is necessary for patients with severe renal impairment. No dosage adjustments based on other identified covariates (age, gender, proteinuria, race) are required for renal allograft patients. No data are available for administration in patients with severe hepatic impairment.
Contraindications	In patients with a known hypersensitivity to the product or any of its components.
Warnings	As part of an immunosuppressive regimen, including cyclosporine, mycophenolate mofetil, and corticosteroids, it may be associated with an increase in mortality. Severe, acute (onset within 24 h) hypersensitivity reactions, including anaphylaxis, have been observed both on initial exposure and following re-exposure.
Adverse Reactions	*Gastrointestinal upsets*: constipation, nausea, vomiting, diarrhea. *Others*: fatigue, tremor, headache, dizziness, increased risk of cellulitis and wound infections, hives, lower-extremity edema, dermatitis. Monitor CBC with differential, ALT, and AST every 2 weeks for the first month then every 4–6 weeks.
Pregnancy Category	C.
Drug Interactions	Safety and effectiveness have been established in pediatric patients from 11 months to 17 years of age. Use in this age group is supported by evidence from adequate and well-controlled studies in adults, with additional pediatric pharmacokinetic data. The following medications have been administered with daclizumab in clinical trials in renal allograft patients with no incremental increase in adverse reactions: cyclosporine, mycophenolate mofetil, ganciclovir, acyclovir, azathioprine, and corticosteroids. Very limited experience exists in these patients with the use of daclizumab concomitantly with tacrolimus, muromonab-CD3, antithymocyte globulin, and antilymphocyte globulin. In renal allograft recipients (n=50) treated with daclizumab and mycophenolate mofetil, no pharmacokinetic interaction between daclizumab and mycophenolic acid, the active metabolite of mycophenolate

mofetil, was observed. However, in a large clinical study in cardiac transplant recipients (n=434), the use of daclizumab as part of an immunosuppression regimen, including cyclosporine, mycophenolate mofetil, and corticosteroids, was associated with an increase in mortality, particularly in patients receiving concomitant antilymphocyte antibody therapy and in patients who developed severe infections.

Dapiprazole Hydrochloride

Brand Name	Rev-Eye.
Class of Drug	Reversal of mydriasis. Alpha-adrenergic-blocking agent.
Indications	Reversal of iatrogenically induced mydriasis produced by adrenergic (phenylephrine) or parasympatholytic (tropicamide) agents. Ophthalmic solution is not indicated for the reduction of IOP or in the treatment of OAG.
Dosage Form	Topical ophthalmic solution 0.5%. Once the ophthalmic solution has been reconstituted, it may be stored at room temperature (59–86°F) for 21 days. Discard any solution that is not clear and colorless.
Dose	2 drops followed 5 min later by an additional 2 drops to reverse diagnostic mydriasis. Should not be used in the same patient more frequently than once per week.
Contraindications	Where constriction is undesirable; such as acute iritis, and in subjects showing hypersensitivity to the product or any of its components.
Warnings	Should not be used in the same patient more frequently than once a week.
Adverse Reactions	In controlled studies, the most frequent reaction was conjunctival injection lasting 20 min in over 80% of patients. Burning on instillation was reported in approximately half of all patients. Reactions occurring in 10–40% of patients included ptosis, lid erythema, lid edema, chemosis, itching, punctate keratitis, corneal edema, brow ache, photophobia, and headaches. Other reactions reported less frequently included dryness of eyes, tearing, and blurring of vision.
Pregnancy Category	B.
Drug Interactions	Negative reports for teratogenicity and impairment of fertility. In animal studies using oral doses 80,000 times the topical dose, increased incidence of liver tumors was found.

Dapsone

Brand Name	Dapsone.
Class of Drug	*Antimicrobial*: sulfonamide/antimicrobial inhibition of folate synthesis; competitively inhibits p-aminobenzoic acid (PABA) in microorganisms, thereby interrupting nucleic acid biosynthesis. *Anti-inflammatory*: inhibits neutrophil chemotaxis.
Indications	*Approved for*: dermatitis herpetiformis; leprosy (all forms except cases of proven resistance). *Other nonophthalmic uses*: malaria, bullous pemphigoid, cicatricial pemphigoid, pemphigus vulgaris, relapsing polychondritis, *Pneumocystis carinii* infection in patients with AIDS, cutaneous leishmaniasis. *Ophthalmic uses*: Cicatricial pemphigoid affecting the conjunctiva (OCP); scleritis associated with relapsing polychondritis; first-line agent for OCP if inflammatory activity is not severe, the disease is not rapidly progressive, and the patient is not glucose6phosphate dehydrogenase (G6PD)-deficient; simple or nodular scleritis associated with relapsing polychondritis; mucocutaneous lesions of Behçet. Ineffective in the treatment of necrotizing scleritis associated with relapsing polychondritis.
Dosage Form	Oral tablets 25 mg, 100 mg.
Dose	25 mg administered two times per day for 1 week then increased to 50 mg two times per day. Maximum of 150 mg/day.
Contraindications	In patients with a history of hypersensitivity to the product or any of its components . Readily crosses the placenta. Use of medication in pregnant women has not been adequately studied. Excreted in human milk in significant quantities; should be avoided in nursing mothers to protect the neonate from potential hemolytic reactions.
Warnings	Patients with G6PD are extremely susceptible to Dapsone-induced hemolysis and methemoglobinemia.*Carcinogenesis/mutagenesis*: Has been found carcinogenic (sarcomagenic) for male rats and female mice causing mesenchymal tumors in the spleen and peritoneum, and thyroid carcinoma in female rats. Not mutagenic with or without microsomal activation in *Salmonella typhimurium* tester strains 1535, 1537, 1538, 98, or 100. *Cutaneous reactions*: especially bullous, include exfoliative dermatitis; probably one of the most serious, though rare, complications of sulfone therapy and are directly due to drug sensitization. Such reactions include toxic erythema, erythema multiforme, toxic epidermal necrolysis, morbilliform and scarlatiniform reactions, urticaria, and erythema nodosum. If new or toxic dermatologic reactions occur, therapy must be promptly discontinued and appropriate therapy instituted.

Caution in patients with G6PD deficiency or methemoglobin reductase deficiency, leukopenia, severe anemia, liver disease, renal insufficiency, and elderly patients.

Adverse Reactions   Methemoglobinemia and dose-related hemolysis (most common). Peripheral neuropathy is a definite but unusual complication in nonleprosy patients. Motor loss is predominant. If muscle weakness appears, dapsone should be withdrawn; recovery on withdrawal is usually substantially complete. Agranulocytosis (relatively rare); sulfone syndrome; rare hypersensitivity reaction manifesting as fever, rash, jaundice, elevated LFTs, and hemolytic anemia can develop at very low doses. Additional adverse reactions include nausea, vomiting, abdominal pains, pancreatitis, vertigo, blurred vision, tinnitus, insomnia, fever, headache, psychosis, phototoxicity, pulmonary eosinophilia, tachycardia, albuminuria, nephrotic syndrome, hypoalbuminemia without proteinuria, renal papillary necrosis, male infertility, drug-induced lupus erythematosus, and infectious mononucleosis-like syndrome. In general, with the exception of the complications of severe anoxia from overdosage (retinal and optic nerve damage, etc.), these reactions have regressed off-drug. Monitoring to determine baseline G6PD levels is mandatory; CBC with differential, ALT, and AST every 2 weeks for the first month then every 4–6 weeks.

Pregnancy Category   C.

Drug Interactions   Children are treated on the same schedule as adults but with correspondingly smaller doses. Generally not considered to have an effect on later growth, development, and functional development of the child. Rifampin lowers dapsone levels 7- to 10-fold by accelerating plasma clearance; in leprosy, this reduction has not required a change in dosage. Folic acid antagonists, such as pyrimethamine, may increase the likelihood of hematologic reactions. A modest interaction has been reported for patients receiving 100 mg dapsone o.d. in combination with trimethoprim 5 mg/kg every 6 h.

Dexamethasone Sodium Phosphate

Brand Name   Decadron.

Class of Drug   Corticosteroid.

Indications   Severe, acute, and chronic allergic and inflammatory processes involving the eye, such as herpes zoster ophthalmicus, iritis, iridocyclitis, chorioretinitis, diffuse posterior uveitis and choroiditis, optic neuritis, sympathetic ophthalmia, anterior segment inflammation, allergic conjunctivitis, keratitis, allergic corneal marginal ulcers.

Dosage Form Decadron phosphate injection 4 mg/ml, 24 mg/ml.

Dose Subconjunctival injection and intraocular injection have been used.

Contraindications In patients with systemic fungal infections or hypersensitivity to the product or any of its components, including sulfites.

Warnings Anaphylactoid and hypersensitivity reactions have been reported. Contains sodium bisulfite, a sulfite that may cause allergic-type reactions, including anaphylactic symptoms and life-threatening or less-severe asthmatic episodes in certain susceptible people. Sulfite sensitivity is seen more frequently in asthmatic than in nonasthmatic people. Corticosteroids may exacerbate systemic fungal infections and therefore should not be used in the presence of such infections unless they are needed to control drug reactions due to amphotericin B. Moreover, there have been cases reported in which concomitant use of amphotericin B and hydrocortisone was followed by cardiac enlargement and congestive failure. In patients on corticosteroid therapy subjected to any unusual stress, increased dosage of rapidly acting corticosteroids before, during, and after the stressful situation is indicated.

Drug-induced secondary adrenocortical insufficiency may result from too rapid withdrawal of corticosteroids and may be minimized by gradual reduction of dosage. This type of relative insufficiency may persist for months after discontinuation of therapy; therefore, in any situation of stress occurring during that period, hormone therapy should be reinstituted. If the patient is receiving steroids already, dosage may have to be increased. Since mineralocorticoid secretion may be impaired, salt and/or a mineralocorticoid should be administered concurrently.

Corticosteroids may mask some signs of infection, and new infections may appear during their use. There may be decreased resistance and inability to localize infection when corticosteroids are used. Moreover, corticosteroids may affect the nitroblue-tetrazolium test for bacterial infection and produce false-negative results. In cerebral malaria, a double-blind trial has shown that the use of corticosteroids is associated with prolongation of coma and a higher incidence of pneumonia and gastrointestinal bleeding. Corticosteroids may activate latent amebiasis. Therefore, it is recommended that latent or active amebiasis be ruled out before initiating corticosteroid therapy in any patient who has spent time in the tropics or any patient with unexplained diarrhea.

Prolonged use of corticosteroids may produce posterior subcapsular cataracts, glaucoma with possible damage to the optic nerves, and may enhance the establishment of secondary ocular infections due to fungi or viruses.

Administration of live virus vaccines, including smallpox, is contraindicated in individuals receiving immunosuppressive doses of corticosteroids. If inactivated viral or bacterial vaccines are administered to individuals receiving immunosuppressive doses of corticosteroids, the expected serum antibody response may not be obtained. However, immunization procedures may be undertaken in patients who are receiving corticosteroids as replacement therapy, e.g., for Addison's disease. Patients who are on drugs that suppress the immune system are more susceptible to infections than healthy individuals. Chickenpox and measles, for example, can have a more serious or even fatal course in nonimmune patients on corticosteroids. In such patients who have not had these diseases, particular care should be taken to avoid exposure. The risk of developing a disseminated infection varies among individuals and can be related to the dose, route, and duration of corticosteroid administration, as well as to the underlying disease. If exposed to chickenpox, prophylaxis with varicella zoster immune globulin (VZIG) may be indicated. If chickenpox develops, treatment with antiviral agents may be considered. If exposed to measles, prophylaxis with immune globulin (IG) may be indicated. (See the respective package inserts for VZIG and IG for complete prescribing information.) Similarly, corticosteroids should be used with great care in patients with a known or suspected Strongyloides (threadworm) infestation. In such patients, corticosteroid-induced immunosuppression may lead to Strongyloides hyperinfection and dissemination with widespread larval migration, often accompanied by severe enterocolitis and potentially fatal gram-negative septicemia.

Use in active tuberculosis should be restricted to those cases of fulminating or disseminated tuberculosis in which the corticosteroid is used for the management of the disease in conjunction with an appropriate antituberculous regimen. If corticosteroids are indicated in patients with latent tuberculosis or tuberculin reactivity, close observation is necessary, as reactivation of the disease may occur. During prolonged corticosteroid therapy, these patients should receive chemoprophylaxis.

Literature reports suggest an apparent association between use of corticosteroids and left ventricular free wall rupture after a recent myocardial infarction; therefore, therapy with corticosteroids should be used with great caution in these patients.

Adverse Reactions   Growth and development of pediatric patients on prolonged corticosteroid therapy should be carefully followed. *Fluid and electrolyte disturbances*: sodium retention, fluid retention, congestive heart failure in susceptible patients, potassium loss, hypokalemic alkalosis, hypertension. *Musculoskeletal*: muscle weakness, steroid myopathy, loss of muscle mass, osteoporosis, vertebral compression fractures, aseptic necrosis of femoral and humeral heads, pathologic fracture of long bones, tendon rupture. *Gastrointestinal*: peptic ulcer with possible subsequent perforation and hemorrhage; perforation of the small and large bowel, particularly in patients with inflammatory bowel disease; pancreatitis, abdominal distention, ulcerative esophagitis. *Dermatologic*: hirsutism, impaired wound healing; thin, fragile skin; petechiae and ecchymoses; erythema; increased sweating; may suppress reactions to skin tests; burning or tingling, especially in the perineal area (after i.v. injection); other cutaneous reactions such as allergic dermatitis, urticaria, angioneurotic edema. *Neurologic*: convulsions, increased intracranial pressure with papilledema (pseudotumor cerebri) usually after treatment, vertigo, headache, psychic disturbances, cerebral palsy in preterm infants. *Endocrine*: menstrual irregularities; development of cushingoid state; suppression of growth in pediatric patients; secondary adrenocortical and pituitary unresponsiveness, particularly in times of stress, as in trauma, surgery, or illness; decreased carbohydrate tolerance. *Manifestations of latent diabetes mellitus*: hyperglycemia, increased requirements for insulin or oral hypoglycemic agents in diabetics. *Ophthalmic*: posterior subcapsular cataracts, increased intraocular pressure, glaucoma, exophthalmos, retinopathy of prematurity. *Metabolic*: negative nitrogen balance due to protein catabolism. *Cardiovascular*: myocardial rupture following recent myocardial infarction, hypertrophic cardiomyopathy in low-birth-weight infants. *Others*: anaphylactoid or hypersensitivity reactions, thromboembolism, weight gain, increased appetite, nausea, malaise, hiccups. *Additional parenteral-related reactions*: rare instances of blindness associated with intralesional therapy around the face and head hyperpigmentation or hypopigmentation, subcutaneous and cutaneous atrophy, sterile abscess, postinjection flare (following intra-articular use), Charcot-like arthropathy.

Pregnancy Category C.

Drug Interactions Mutual inhibition of metabolism occurs with concurrent use of cyclosporin and corticosteroids; therefore, it is possible that adverse events associated with the individual use of either drug may be more apt to occur. Drugs that induce hepatic enzymes, such as phenobarbital, phenytoin, and rifampin, may increase the clearance of corticosteroids. Drugs such as troleandomycin and ketoconazole may inhibit the metabolism of corticosteroids and thus decrease its clearance. Corticosteroids may increase the clearance of chronic high-dose aspirin; this could lead to decreased salicylate serum levels or increase the risk of salicylate toxicity when corticosteroid is withdrawn; aspirin should be used cautiously in conjunction with corticosteroids in patients suffering from hypoprothrombinemia. The effect of corticosteroids on oral anticoagulants is variable. There are reports of enhanced as well as diminished effects of anticoagulant when given concurrently with corticosteroids. Therefore, coagulation indices should be monitored to maintain the desired anticoagulant effect.

Brand Name Decadron Phosphate; Maxidex.

Class of Drug Corticosteroid.

Indications Steroid-responsive inflammatory conditions of the palpebral and bulbar conjunctiva, cornea, and anterior segment of the globe, such as allergic conjunctivitis, acne rosacea, superficial punctate keratitis, herpes zoster keratitis, iritis, cyclitis, selected infective conjunctivitis when the inherent hazard of steroid use is accepted to obtain an advisable diminution in edema and inflammation; corneal injury from chemical or thermal burns or penetration of foreign bodies.

Dosage Form Topical: *Ophthalmic solution* 0.1%. *Ophthalmic ointment* 0.05%.

Dose *Solution*: 1–2 drops into the conjunctival sac every hour during the day and every 2 h during the night as initial therapy. *Ointment*: thin coat three to four times a day. When a favorable response is observed, reduce dosage. Duration of treatment will vary with type of lesion.

Contraindications See »Decadron.« Epithelial herpes simplex keratitis (dendritic keratitis); acute infectious stages of vaccinia, varicella, and many other viral diseases of the cornea and conjunctiva; mycobacterial infection of the eye; fungal diseases of ocular structures; hypersensitivity to the product or any of its components, including sulfites.

Warnings See »Decadron.« Prolonged use may result in ocular hypertension and/or glaucoma and posterior subcapsular cataract formation and suppress the host response, thus increasing the hazard of secondary ocular infections. In diseases causing thinning of the cornea or sclera, perforations have been known to occur with the use of topical corticosteroids. In acute purulent conditions of the eye, corticosteroids may mask infection or enhance existing infection. If these products are used for 10 days or longer, IOP should be routinely monitored even though it may be difficult in children and uncooperative patients. Employment of corticosteroid medication in the treatment of herpes simplex other than epithelial herpes simplex keratitis, in which it is contraindicated, requires great caution; periodic slit-lamp microscopy is essential.

Adverse Reactions Glaucoma with optic nerve damage; visual acuity and field defects; posterior subcapsular cataract formation; secondary ocular infection from pathogens, including herpes simplex; perforation of the globe. *Rarely*: filtering blebs have been reported when topical steroids have been used following cataract surgery; stinging or burning may occur. Sodium bisulfite, the preservative in Decadron, is a sulfite that may cause allergic-type reactions, including anaphylactic symptoms and life-threatening or less-severe asthmatic episodes in certain susceptible people. The overall prevalence of sulfite sensitivity in the general population is unknown and probably low. Sulfite sensitivity is seen more frequently in asthmatic than in nonasthmatic people.

Pregnancy Category C.

Drug Interactions Corticosteroids have been found to be teratogenic in animal studies. There are no adequate and well-controlled studies in pregnant women. It is not known whether topical administration of corticosteroids could result in sufficient systemic absorption to produce detectable quantities in human milk.

Dexamethasone and Antibiotic

Brand Name Maxitrol (neomycin, polymyxin B sulfate, dexamethasone).

Class of Drug Steroid/antibiotic. *Neomycin*: inhibits protein synthesis by binding with ribosomal RNA. *Polymyxin B*: increases the permeability of the bacterial cell membrane.

Indications Steroid-responsive inflammatory conditions of the palpebral and bulbar conjunctiva, cornea, and anterior segment of the globe where the inherent risk of steroid use in certain infective conjunctivitides is accepted to obtain a diminution in edema and inflammation. Also in chronic anterior uveitis and corneal injury from chemical radiation or thermal burns or penetration of foreign bodies. The particular anti-infective drug in this product is active against the following common bacterial eye pathogens: *S. aureus, E. coli, H. influenzae, Klebsiella/Enterobacter* spp., *Neisseria* spp., and *P. aeruginosa*. This product does not provide adequate coverage against *S. marcescens* and streptococci, including *S. pneumoniae*.

Dosage Form Ophthalmic suspension or ointment: each milliliter of suspension or each gram of ointment contains neomycin sulfate equivalent to neomycin 3.5 mg, polymyxin B sulfate 10,000 U, and dexamethasone 0.1%.

Dose *Suspension*: 1–2 drops topically in the conjunctival sac(s). In severe disease, drops may be used hourly, being tapered to discontinuation as the inflammation subsides. In mild disease, drops may be used up to four to six times per day. *Ointment*: small amount into the conjunctival sac(s) up to three to four times per day, or may be used adjunctively with drops at bedtime.

Contraindications Epithelial herpes simplex keratitis (dendritic keratitis), vaccinia, varicella, and many other viral diseases of the cornea and conjunctiva. Mycobacterial infection of the eye. Fungal diseases of ocular structures. Hypersensitivity to the product or any of its components.

Warnings

Prolonged use may result in ocular hypertension and/or glaucoma and posterior subcapsular cataract formation. Prolonged use may suppress the host response and thus increase the hazard of secondary ocular infections. In those diseases causing thinning of the cornea or sclera, perforations have been known to occur with the use of topical corticosteroids. In acute purulent conditions of the eye, corticosteroids may mask infection or enhance existing infection. If these products are used for 10 days or longer, IOP should be routinely monitored even though it may be difficult in children and uncooperative patients. Products containing neomycin sulfate may cause cutaneous sensitization. Employment of steroid medication in the treatment of herpes simplex requires great caution. The possibility of persistent fungal infections of the cornea should be considered after prolonged steroid dosing.

Adverse Reactions

Hypersensitivity and localized ocular toxicity, including lid itching and swelling, and conjunctival erythema. Reactions due to the steroid component are elevation of IOP with possible development of glaucoma, and infrequent optic nerve damage; posterior subcapsular cataract formation; delayed wound healing. The development of secondary infection has occurred after use of combinations containing steroids and antimicrobials. Fungal infections of the cornea are particularly prone to develop coincidentally with long-term applications of steroid. The possibility of fungal invasion must be considered in any persistent corneal ulceration where steroid treatment has been used.

Pregnancy Category

C.

Drug Interactions

Corticosteroids have been found to be teratogenic in animal studies. There are no adequate and well-controlled studies in pregnant women. It is not known whether topical administration of corticosteroids could result in sufficient systemic absorption to produce detectable quantities in human mild. Safety and effectiveness in pediatric patients younger than 2 years of age have not been established.

Brand Name

NeoDecadron (neomycin sulfate-dexamethasone sodium phosphate).

Class of Drug

Steroid/antibiotic. Neomycin: inhibits protein synthesis by binding with ribosomal RNA.

Indications

Use of a combination drug with an anti-infective component is indicated where the risk of infection is high or where there is an expectation that potentially dangerous numbers of bacteria will be present in the eye. The particular anti-infective drug in this product is active against the following common bacterial eye pathogens: *S. aureus, E. coli, H. influenzae, Klebsiella/Enterobacter* spp., *Neisseria* spp. The product does not provide adequate coverage against: *P. aeruginosa, S. marcescens,* or streptococci, including *S. pneumoniae.*

Dosage Form
Sterile ophthalmic solution: each milliliter contains 3.5 mg neomycin sulfate and 1 mg (0.1%) dexamethasone sodium phosphate.

Dose
1–2 drops into the conjunctival sac every hour during the day and every 2 h during the night as initial therapy. When a favorable response is observed, reduce dosage. Not more than 20 ml should be prescribed initially, and the prescription should not be refilled without further evaluation.

Contraindications
Most viral diseases of the cornea and conjunctiva, including epithelial herpes simplex keratitis (dendritic keratitis), vaccinia, varicella. Mycobacterial infection of the eye and fungal diseases of ocular structures. In individuals with a known or suspected hypersensitivity to the product or any of its components, including sulfites, and to other corticosteroids (hypersensitivity to the antibiotic component occurs at a higher rate than for other components).

Warnings
If this product is used for 10 days or longer, IOP should be routinely monitored even though it may be difficult in children and uncooperative patients. Corticosteroids should be used with caution in the presence of ocular hypertension and/or glaucoma. The use of corticosteroids after cataract surgery may delay healing and increase the incidence of filtering blebs. Neomycin sulfate may occasionally cause cutaneous sensitization. If any reaction indicating such sensitivity is observed, discontinue use. NeoDecadron contains sodium bisulfite, a sulfite that may cause allergic-type reactions, including anaphylactic symptoms and life-threatening or less-severe asthmatic episodes in certain susceptible people. Overall prevalence of sulfite sensitivity in the general population is unknown and probably low. Sulfite sensitivity is seen more frequently in asthmatic than in nonasthmatic people.

Adverse Reactions
Reactions due to the steroid component are as above. Reactions occurring most often from the presence of the anti-infective ingredient are allergic sensitizations. Reactions due to the corticosteroid component in decreasing order of frequency are elevation of IOP with possible development of glaucoma and infrequent optic nerve damage; posterior subcapsular cataract formation; delayed wound healing. Development of secondary infection has occurred after use of combinations containing corticosteroids and antimicrobials. Fungal and viral infections of the cornea are particularly prone to develop coincidentally with long-term application of a corticosteroid. The possibility of fungal invasion must be considered in any persistent corneal ulceration where corticosteroid treatment has been used.

Pregnancy Category
C.

Drug Interactions
See »Maxitrol«

Brand Name   TobraDex.

Class of Drug   Steroid/antibiotic. Disrupting bacterial protein synthesis leading to altered cell membrane permeability and progressive disruption of the cell envelop.

Indications   The use of a combination drug with an anti-infective component is indicated where the risk of superficial ocular infection is high or where there is an expectation that potentially dangerous numbers of bacteria will be present in the eye and postoperatively when a combination of the two medications may increase compliance. Tobramycin in this product is active against the following common bacterial eye pathogens: staphylococci, including *S. aureus* and *S. epidermidis* (coagulase-positive and coagulase-negative), including penicillin-resistant strains; streptococci, including some of the group A beta-hemolytic species, some nonhemolytic species, and some *S. pneumoniae*; *P. aeruginosa*; *E. coli;*, *K. pneumoniae*; *E. aerogenes*; *P. mirabilis*; *M. morganii*; most *P. vulgaris* strains; *H. influenzae* and *Haemophilus aegyptius*; *M. lacunata*; *A. calcoaceticus*; some *Neisseria* spp.

Dosage Form   Ophthalmic suspension or ointment: tobramycin 0.3%, dexamethasone 0.1%.

Dose   *Suspension*: 1–2 drops every 4–6 h. During the initial 24–48 h, the dosage may be increased to 1 or 2 drops every 2 h. Frequency should be decreased gradually as warranted by improvement in clinical signs. *Ointment*: small amount [1-cm (approx. ½-in.) ribbon] up to three or four times per day.

Contraindications Epithelial herpes simplex keratitis (dendritic keratitis), vaccinia, varicella, and many other viral diseases of the cornea and conjunctiva. Mycobacterial infection of the eye. Fungal diseases of ocular structures. Hypersensitivity to the product or any of its components.

Warnings   Sensitivity to topically applied aminoglycosides may occur in some patients. If a sensitivity reaction does occur, discontinue use. Prolonged use of steroids may result in glaucoma, with damage to the optic nerve, defects in visual acuity and fields of vision, and posterior subcapsular cataract formation. IOP should be routinely monitored even though it may be difficult in pediatric and uncooperative patients. Prolonged use may suppress the host response and thus increase the hazard of secondary ocular infections. In those diseases causing thinning of the cornea or sclera, perforations have been known to occur with the use of topical steroids. In acute purulent conditions of the eye, steroids may mask infection or enhance existing infection. Cross-sensitivity to other aminoglycoside antibiotics may occur.

Adverse Reactions Most frequent to topical ocular tobramycin (Tobrex) are hypersensitivity and localized ocular toxicity, including lid itching and swelling, and conjunctival erythema. These reactions occur in less than 4% of patients. Similar reactions may occur with the topical use of other aminoglycoside antibiotics. Other adverse reactions have not been reported; however, if topical ocular tobramycin is administered concomitantly with systemic aminoglycoside antibiotics, care should be taken to monitor the total serum concentration. Reactions due to the steroid component are elevation of IOP with possible development of glaucoma, and infrequent optic nerve damage; posterior subcapsular cataract formation; delayed wound healing. The development of secondary infection has occurred after use of combinations containing steroids and antimicrobials. Fungal infections of the cornea are particularly prone to develop coincidentally with long-term applications of steroids. The possibility of fungal invasion must be considered in any persistent corneal ulceration where steroid treatment has been used.

Secondary bacterial ocular infection following suppression of host responses also occurs.

Pregnancy Category	C.
Drug Interactions	»See Maxitrol«

Dextran 70

Brand Name	Advanced Relief Visine
Class of Drug	Lubricant/redness reliever.
Indications	Relief of redness of the eye due to minor eye irritations and as a protectant against further irritation or to relieve dryness of the eye.
Dosage Form	Topical ophthalmic solution. Dextran 70 0.1%, polyethylene glycol 400 1%, and povidone 1% as lubricants; tetrahydrozoline HCl 0.05% as redness reliever.
Dose	1 or 2 drops to affected eye(s) up to four times per day.
Contraindications	See »Bion Tears.«
Warnings	Ask a doctor before use if you have NAG. Pupils may become enlarged temporarily. Overuse may cause more eye redness.
Pregnancy Category	C.

Brand Name	Bion Tears.
Class of Drug	Lubricant eye drops.
Indications	Relief of dry-eye symptoms.
Dosage Form	DuaSorb; water-soluble polymeric system containing dextran 70 0.1% and hydroxypropyl methylcellulose 2910 0.3%. Preservative free.
Dose	1 or 2 drops to affected eye(s) as needed. To ensure optimal effectiveness once the pouch is opened, the containers inside the pouch must be used within 4 days (96 h).

Contraindications	In patients with a known hypersensitivity to the product or any of its components.
Warnings	If patient experiences eye pain, changes in vision, continued redness, or irritation of the eye, or if the condition worsens or persists for more than 72 h, patient should discontinue use and consult a doctor. If solution changes color or becomes cloudy, do not use.
Pregnancy Category	C.
Brand Name	Tears Naturale Forte.
Class of Drug	Lubricant eye drops.
Indications	Temporary relief of burning and irritation due to dryness of the eye and as a protectant against further irritation. Temporary relief of discomfort due to minor irritations of the eye or to exposure to wind or sun.
Dosage Form	Topical ophthalmic solution. Dextran 70 0.1%, glycerin 0.2%, hydroxypropyl methylcellulose 0.3%. Preservative: Polyquad (polyquaternium-1) 0.001%.
Dose	1 or 2 drops to affected eye(s) as needed.
Contraindications	See »Bion Tears.«
Warnings	See »Bion Tears.«
Pregnancy Category	C.
Brand Name	Tear Naturale Free.
Class of Drug	Lubricant eye drops.
Indications	See »Bion Tears.«
Dosage Form	Topical ophthalmic solution. DuaSorb, water soluble polymeric system containing dextran 70 0.1% and hydroxypropyl methylcellulose 2910 0.3%. Preservative free.
Dose	1 or 2 drops to affected eye(s) as needed. Discard container 12 h after opening.
Contraindications	See »Bion Tears.«
Warnings	See »Bion Tears.«
Pregnancy Category	C.

Dichlorphenamide

Brand Name	Daranide.
Class of Drug	Glaucoma. CAI (sulfonamide).
Indications	Adjunctive treatment of chronic, simple (open-angle) glaucoma; secondary glaucoma; preoperatively in acute ACG where delay of surgery is desired in order to lower IOP.
Dosage Form	Oral tablets 50 mg.
Dose	Dosage must be adjusted carefully to meet the requirements of the individual patient. A priming dose of 100–200 mg (2–4

tablets) is suggested for adults, followed by 100 mg (2 tablets) every 12 h until the desired response has been obtained. Recommended maintenance dosage for adults is 25–50 mg once to three times per day.

Contraindications

In hepatic insufficiency, renal failure, adrenocortical insufficiency, hyperchloremic acidosis, or conditions in which serum levels of sodium or potassium are depressed. Should not be used in patients with severe pulmonary obstruction who are unable to increase their alveolar ventilation since their acidosis may be increased; patients who are hypersensitive to the product or any of its components.

Warnings

Potassium excretion is increased by Daranide, and hypokalemia may develop with brisk diuresis when severe cirrhosis is present or during concomitant use of steroids or adrenocorticotropic hormone (ACTH). Interference with adequate oral electrolyte intake will also contribute to hypokalemia. Hypokalemia can sensitize or exaggerate the response of the heart to the toxic effects of digitalis (e.g., increased ventricular irritability). Hypokalemia may be avoided or treated by use of potassium supplements, such as foods with high potassium content. Daranide should be used with caution in patients with respiratory acidosis.

Adverse Reactions

Certain side-effects characteristic of CAIs may occur, particularly with increasing doses (see »Acetazolamide«). Most common effects include gastrointestinal disturbances (anorexia, nausea, and vomiting), drowsiness, and paresthesias. Included in the listing which follows are some adverse reactions which have not been reported with Daranide. However, pharmacological similarities among the CAIs make it advisable to consider the following reactions when dichlorphenamide is administered. *CNS/psychiatric*: ataxia, tremor, tinnitus, headache, weakness, nervousness, globus hystericus, lassitude, depression, confusion, disorientation, dizziness. *Gastrointestinal*: constipation, hepatic insufficiency. *Metabolic*: loss of weight, metabolic acidosis, electrolyte imbalance (hypokalemia, hyperchloremia), hyperuricemia. *Hypersensitivity*: skin eruptions, pruritus, fever. *Hematologic*: leukopenia, agranulocytosis, thrombocytopenia. *Genitourinary*: urinary frequency, renal colic, renal calculi, phosphaturia.

Pregnancy Category

C.

Drug Interactions

Should not be used in women of childbearing age or in pregnancy, especially during the first trimester, unless the potential benefits outweigh the potential risks. Caution is advised in patients receiving concomitant high-dose aspirin and carbonic anhydrase inhibitors, as anorexia, tachypnea, lethargy, and coma have been rarely reported due to a possible drug interaction. Safety and effectiveness in pediatric patients have not been established.

Diclofenac Sodium

Brand Name	Voltaren Ophthalmic.
Class of Drug	NSAID.
Indications	Postoperative inflammation in patients who have undergone cataract extraction. Temporary relief of pain and photophobia in patients undergoing corneal refractive surgery. Cystoid macular edema (off-label use).
Dosage Form	Topical ophthalmic solution 0.1%.
Dose	*Cataract surgery*: 1 drop four times per day beginning 24 h after surgery and continuing throughout the first 2 weeks of the postoperative period. *Corneal refractive surgery*: 1–2 drops to the operative eye within the hour prior to surgery; within 15 min after surgery, 1–2 drops then continued four times per day up to 3 days. *Cystoid macular edema*: 1 drop four times per day (off-label use).
Contraindications	In patients who are hypersensitive to the product or any of its components .
Warnings	Refractive stability of patients undergoing corneal refractive procedures and treated with Voltaren has not been established. Patients should be monitored for a year following use in this setting. With some NSAIDs, there exists the potential for increased bleeding time due to interference with thrombocyte aggregation. There have been reports that ocularly applied NSAIDs can cause increased bleeding of ocular tissues (including hyphemas) in conjunction with ocular surgery. There is the potential for cross-sensitivity to acetylsalicylic acid, phenylacetic acid derivatives, and other nonsteroidal anti-inflammatory agents. Therefore, caution should be used when treating individuals who have previously exhibited sensitivities to these drugs. All topical NSAIDs may slow or delay healing. Topical corticosteroids are also known to slow or delay healing. Concomitant use of topical NSAIDs and topical steroids may increase the potential for healing problems. Use of topical NSAIDs may result in keratitis. In some susceptible patients, continued use of topical NSAIDs may result in epithelial breakdown, corneal thinning, corneal infiltrates, corneal erosion, corneal ulceration, and corneal perforation. These events may be sight threatening. Patients with evidence of corneal epithelial breakdown should immediately discontinue use of topical NSAIDs and should be closely monitored for corneal health. Postmarketing experience with topical NSAIDs suggests that patients experiencing complicated ocular surgeries, corneal denervation, corneal epithelial defects, diabetes mellitus, ocular surface disease (e.g., dry-eye syndrome), rheumatoid arthritis, or repeat ocular surgeries within a short period of time may be at increased risk for corneal adverse events, which may become sight threatening. Topical NSAIDs should be used with caution in these patients.

Postmarketing experience with topical NSAIDs also suggests that use more than 24 h prior to surgery or beyond 14 days post surgery may increase patient risk for occurrence and severity of corneal adverse events. Results from clinical studies indicate that Voltaren has no significant effect upon ocular pressure. However, elevations in IOP may occur following cataract surgery.

Adverse Reactions

Identified during postmarketing use of topical diclofenac sodium ophthalmic solution 0.1% in clinical practice: corneal erosion, corneal infiltrates, corneal perforation, corneal thinning, corneal ulceration, epithelial breakdown, superficial punctate keratitis.*Ocular*: 15% of patients across studies experienced transient burning and stinging; up to 28% of patients in cataract surgery studies reported keratitis although in many of these cases keratitis was initially noted prior to the initiation of treatment; ~15% of patients undergoing cataract surgery reported elevated IOP; ~30% of case studies undergoing incisional refractive surgery complained of lacrimation; ~5% or less of patients experienced: abnormal vision, acute elevated IOP, blurred vision, conjunctivitis, corneal deposits, corneal edema, corneal opacity, corneal lesions, discharge, eyelid swelling, injection, iritis, irritation, itching, lacrimation disorder, ocular allergy. *Systemic*: 3% or less of patients reported abdominal pain, asthenia, chills, dizziness, facial edema, fever, headache, insomnia, nausea, pain, rhinitis, viral infection, vomiting.

Pregnancy Category

C.

Drug Interactions

Carcinogenesis, mutagenesis, impairment of fertility: Long-term carcinogenicity studies in rats given Voltaren in oral doses up to 2 mg/kg per day (approximately the human oral dose) revealed no significant increases in tumor incidence. There was a slight increase in benign rat mammary fibroadenomas in mid-dose females (high-dose females had excessive mortality), but the increase was not significant for this common rat tumor. A 2-year carcinogenicity study conducted in mice employing oral Voltaren up to 2 mg/kg per day did not reveal any oncogenic potential. Did not show mutagenic potential in various mutagenicity studies, including the Ames test. Administered to male and female rats at 4 mg/kg per day did not affect fertility. *Nonteratogenic effects*: because of the known effects of prostaglandin biosynthesis-inhibiting drugs on the fetal cardiovascular system (closure of ductus arteriosus), use during late pregnancy should be avoided.

Dipivefrin Hydrochloride

Brand Name	Propine.
Class of Drug	Glaucoma. Converted to epinephrine inside the human eye by enzyme hydrolysis; the liberated epinephrine is an adrenergic agonist.
Indications	OAG. Patients responding inadequately to other antiglaucoma therapy may respond to addition of dipivefrin hydrochloride.
Dosage Form	Topical ophthalmic solution 0.1%.
Dose	Usual dosage is 1 drop in the eye(s) every 12 h.
Contraindications	In patients who are hypersensitive the product or any of its components . Should not be used in patients with NAG since any dilation of the pupil may predispose the patient to an attack of ACG.
Warnings	Macular edema has been shown to occur in up to 30% of aphakic patients treated with epinephrine. Discontinuation of epinephrine generally results in reversal of the maculopathy.
Adverse Reactions	*Cardiovascular:* tachycardia, arrhythmias, and hypertension have been reported with ocular administration of epinephrine. *Local:* most frequent side effects reported with dipivefrin hydrochloride alone were hyperemia in 6.5% of patients and burning and stinging in 6%. Follicular conjunctivitis, eye pain, mydriasis, blurry vision, eye pruritus, headache, and allergic reaction have been reported. Epinephrine therapy can lead to adrenochrome deposits in the conjunctiva and cornea.
Pregnancy Category	B.
Drug Interactions	*Animal studies:* rabbit studies indicated a dose-related incidence of meibomian gland retention cysts following topical administration of both dipivefrin hydrochloride and epinephrine.

Dorzolamide Hydrochloride

Brand Name	Cosopt.
Class of Drug	CAI (sulfonamide) and beta-adrenergic-blocking agents.
Indications	Reduction of elevated IOP in patients with OAG or ocular hypertension who are insufficiently responsive to beta-blockers (failed to achieve target IOP determined after multiple measurements over time). IOP-lowering effect of Cosopt two times per day was slightly less than that seen with concomi-

	tant administration of 0.5% timolol two times per day and 2.0% dorzolamide three times per day
Dosage Form	Topical ophthalmic solution: each milliliter contains 20 mg dorzolamide hydrochloride and 5 mg timolol maleate.
Dose	1 drop two times per day
Contraindications	In patients with bronchial asthma, history of bronchial asthma, severe chronic obstructive pulmonary disease, sinus bradycardia, second- or third-degree AV block, overt cardiac failure, cardiogenic shock, or hypersensitivity to the product or any of its components.
Warnings	Contains dorzolamide, a sulfonamide; and timolol maleate, a beta-adrenergic-blocking agent. Although administered topically, it is absorbed systemically (see »Timolol Maleate« and »Dorzolamide«).
Adverse Reactions	Approximately 5% of all patients discontinued therapy because of adverse reactions. *Most frequently reported*: taste perversion (bitter, sour, or unusual taste) or ocular burning and/or stinging (up to 30% of patients); conjunctival hyperemia, blurred vision, superficial punctate keratitis, or eye itching (between 5–15% of patients); abdominal pain, back pain, blepharitis, bronchitis, cloudy vision, conjunctival discharge, conjunctival edema, conjunctival follicles, conjunctival injection, conjunctivitis, corneal erosion, corneal staining, cortical lens opacity, cough, dizziness, dryness of eyes, dyspepsia, eye debris, eye discharge, eye pain, eye tearing, eyelid edema, eyelid erythema, eyelid exudate/scales, eyelid pain or discomfort, foreign-body sensation, glaucomatous cupping, headache, hypertension, influenza, lens nucleus coloration, lens opacity, nausea, nuclear lens opacity, pharyngitis, postsubcapsular cataract, sinusitis, URTI, UTI, visual field defect, vitreous detachment (1–5% of patients). The following occurred in clinical practice: bradycardia, cardiac failure, cerebral vascular accident, chest pain, depression, diarrhea, dry mouth, dyspnea, hypotension, iridocyclitis, myocardial infarction, nasal congestion, paresthesia, photophobia, respiratory failure, skin rashes, urolithiasis, and vomiting. Other adverse reactions that have been reported with the individual components are listed separately under »Dorzolamide« and »Timolol Maleate.«
Pregnancy Category	C.
Drug Interactions	*CAIs*: Potential for additive effect on the known systemic effects of CAIs in patients receiving an oral carbonic anhydrase inhibitor and Cosopt; concomitant administration with oral CAIs is not recommended. *Acid-base disturbances*: although acid-base and electrolyte disturbances were not reported in clinical trials with dorzolamide hydrochloride ophthalmic solution, these disturbances have been reported with oral CAIs and have, in some instances, resulted in drug interactions (e.g., toxicity associated with high-dose salicylate therapy). Potential for such drug interactions should be considered in

patients receiving Cosopt. *Beta-adrenergic-blocking agents*: Patients receiving a beta-adrenergic-blocking agent orally and Cosopt should be observed for potential additive effects of beta blockade, both systemic and on IOP. Concomitant use of two topical beta-adrenergic-blocking agents is not recommended. *Calcium antagonists*: Caution should be used in the coadministration of beta-adrenergic-blocking agents, such as Cosopt, and oral or i.v. calcium antagonists because of possible AV conduction disturbances, left ventricular failure, and hypotension. In patients with impaired cardiac function, co-administration should be avoided. *Catecholamine-depleting drugs*: Close observation is recommended when a beta-blocker is administered to patients receiving catecholamine-depleting drugs, such as reserpine, because of possible additive effects and the production of hypotension and/or marked bradycardia, which may result in vertigo, syncope, or postural hypotension. *Digitalis and calcium antagonists*: concomitant use of beta-adrenergic-blocking agents with digitalis and calcium antagonists may have additive effects in prolonging AV conduction time. *Quinidine*: potentiated systemic beta blockade (e.g., decreased heart rate) has been reported during combined treatment with quinidine and timolol, possibly because quinidine inhibits the metabolism of timolol via the P-450 enzyme, CYP2D6. *Clonidine*: oral beta-adrenergic-blocking agents may exacerbate the rebound hypertension, which can follow withdrawal of clonidine; there have been no reports of exacerbation of rebound hypertension with ophthalmic timolol maleate.

Brand Name	Trusopt.
Class of Drug	CAI (sulfonamide).
Indications	Elevated IOP in patients with ocular hypertension or OAG.
Dosage Form	Topical ophthalmic solution 2%.
Dose	1 drop to the eye(s) three times per day
Contraindications	In patients who are hypersensitive to the product or any of its components .
Warnings	Trusopt is a sulfonamide and although administered topically is absorbed systemically. Therefore, the same types of adverse reactions attributable to sulfonamides may occur. Fatalities have occurred, although rarely, due to severe reactions to sulfonamides, including Stevens–Johnson syndrome, toxic epidermal necrolysis, fulminant hepatic necrosis, agranulocytosis, aplastic anemia, and other blood dyscrasias. Sensitization may recur when a sulfonamide is readministered irrespective of the route of administration. If signs of serious reactions or hypersensitivity occur, discontinue the use of this preparation. Has not been studied in patients with severe renal impairment (CrCl <30 ml/min); because Trusopt and its metabolite are excreted predominantly by the kidney, it is not recommended in such patients. Has not been studied in patients with he-

patic impairment and should therefore be used with caution in such patients. There is a potential for an additive effect on the known systemic effects of carbonic anhydrase inhibition in patients receiving an oral carbonic anhydrase inhibitor and Trusopt. Concomitant administration with oral carbonic anhydrase inhibitors is not recommended. Choroidal detachment has been reported with administration of aqueous suppressant therapy (e.g., dorzolamide) after filtration procedures.

Adverse Reactions

Most frequent: ocular burning, stinging, or discomfort immediately following ocular administration (approximately one-third of patients). Bitter taste following administration (approximately one-quarter of patients). Superficial punctate keratitis (10–15% of patients), and signs and symptoms of ocular allergic reaction (approximately 10% of patients). *Less frequent*: conjunctivitis and lid reactions, blurred vision, eye redness, tearing, dryness, and photophobia (approximately 1–5% of patients). *Other ocular and systemic events*: include headache, nausea, asthenia/fatigue, and, rarely, skin rashes, urolithiasis, and iridocyclitis (reported infrequently).

The following occurred either at low incidence (<1%) during clinical trials or have been reported during use in clinical practice: signs and symptoms of systemic allergic reactions, including angioedema, bronchospasm, pruritus, and urticaria; dizziness; paresthesia; ocular pain; transient myopia; choroidal detachment following filtration surgery; eyelid crusting; dyspnea; contact dermatitis; epistaxis; dry mouth; throat irritation.

Pregnancy Category
C.

Drug Interactions
Although acid-base and electrolyte disturbances were not reported in clinical trials, these disturbances have been reported with oral carbonic anhydrase inhibitors and have, in some instances, resulted in drug interactions (e.g., toxicity associated with high-dose salicylate therapy). Therefore, the potential for such drug interactions should be considered.

Echothiophate Iodide

Brand Name   Phospholine Iodide.

Class of Drug   Parasympathomimetic, miotic. Cholinesterase inhibitor.

Indications   *Glaucoma*: OAG or ACG after iridectomy or where surgery is refused or contraindicated; certain nonuveitic secondary glaucoma, especially glaucoma following cataract surgery. *Accommodative esotropia*: concomitant esotropias with a significant accommodative component.

Dosage Form   Topical ophthalmic solution: 0.03%, 0.06%, 0.125%, 0.25%.

Dose   *Glaucoma*: brief trial of 0.03% two times per day before higher strengths are used. *Accommodative esotropia diagnosis*: 1 drop of 0.125% may be instilled once per day in both eyes on retiring for a period of 2 or 3 weeks. If the esotropia is accommodative, a favorable response will usually be noted, which may begin within a few hours. *Accommodative esotropia treatment*: Echothiophate iodide is prescribed at the lowest concentration and frequency, which gives satisfactory results. After the initial period of treatment for diagnostic purposes, the schedule may be reduced to 0.125% every other day or 0.06% every day. These dosages can often be gradually lowered as treatment progresses. The 0.03% strength has proven to be effective in some cases. The maximum usually recommended dosage is 0.125% once per day although more intensive therapy has been used for short periods.

Contraindications   Active uveal inflammation; most cases of ACG due to the possibility of increasing angle block (gonioscopy is recommended prior to initiation of therapy); hypersensitivity to the product or any of its components.

Warnings   Succinylcholine should be administered only with great caution, if at all, prior to or during general anesthesia to patients receiving anticholinesterase medication because of possible respiratory or cardiovascular collapse. Caution should be observed in treating glaucoma with echothiophate iodide in patients who are at the same time undergoing treatment with systemic anticholinesterase medications for myasthenia gravis because of possible adverse additive effects.

Adverse Reactions   Although the relationship, if any, of retinal detachment to the administration of echothiophate iodide has not been established, retinal detachment has been reported in a few cases during the use of echothiophate iodide in adult patients without a previous history of this disorder. Stinging, burning, lacrimation, lid-muscle twitching, conjunctival and ciliary redness, and brow ache-induced myopia with visual blurring may occur. Activation of latent iritis or uveitis may occur. Iris cysts may form, and if treatment is continued, may enlarge and obscure vision. This occurrence is more frequent in children. The cysts usually shrink upon discontinuance of the medication and reduction in strength of the drops or frequency of instillation. Rarely, cysts may rupture or break free into the aqueous. Regular examinations are advisable when the drug is being prescribed for the treatment of accommodative esotropia. Prolonged use may cause conjunctival thickening or obstruction of nasolacrimal canals. Lens opacities occurring in patients under treatment for glaucoma with echothiophate iodide have been reported. Routine examinations should accompany clinical use of the drug. Paradoxical increase in IOP may follow anticholinesterase instillation. This may be alleviated by prescribing a sympathomimetic mydriatic, such as phenylephrine. Cardiac irregularities.

Pregnancy Category   C.

Drug Interaction   Potentiates othercholinesterase inhibitors, such as succinylcholine or organophosphate, and carbamate insecticides. Patients undergoing systemic anticholinesterase treatment should be warned of the possible additive effects.

Edetate Disodium (EDTA, Ethylenediamine Tetra Acetate)

Brand Name   Disotate; Endrate; Meritate.

Class of Drug   Chelating agent.

Indications   Band keratopathy.

Dosage Form   Ampule 150 mg/ml (15% solution), 20 ml. Dilute 2 ml of 15% of EDTA solution with 8 ml of normal saline. This gives a 3% mixture.

Dose   Anesthetize the eye with a topical anesthesia. Débride the corneal epithelium with a sterile scalpel or a sterile cotton-tipped applicator dipped in cocaine 4%. Wipe a cellulose sponge or cotton swab saturated with the 3% EDTA solution over the band keratopathy until the calcium clears (which may take 10–30 min).

Contraindications   Known allergy or sensitivity to the drug.

Warnings   The following may apply to systemic administration: Because of the possibility of inducing an electrolyteimbalance during treatment, appropriate laboratory determinations and studies to evaluate the status of cardiac function should be performed.

Pregnancy Category C.

Drug Interactions   Theoxalate method of determining serum calcium tends to give low readings in the presence of edetate disodium.

Emedastine Difumarate

Brand Name   Emadine.
Class of Drug   Selective histamine H1 antagonist.
Indications   Allergic conjunctivitis.
Dosage Form   Topical ophthalmic solution 0.05%.
Dose   1 drop up to four times per day.
Contraindications   In patients with a known hypersensitivity to the product or
                         any of its components.
Warnings   Somnolence and malaise have been reported following daily
                         oral administration. Oral ingestion of the contents of a 15 ml
                         drop-tainer would be equivalent to 7.5 mg. In case of overdo-
                         se, treatment is symptomatic and supportive.
Adverse Reactions   In controlled clinical studies lasting for 42 days, the most fre-
                         quent adverse reaction was headache (11%). Less than 5%
                         of patients experienced the following events, of which some
                         were similar to the underlying disease being studied: abnor-
                         mal dreams, asthenia, bad taste, blurred vision, burning or
                         stinging, corneal infiltrates, corneal staining, dermatitis, dis-
                         comfort, dry eye, foreign-body sensation, hyperemia, kerati-
                         tis, pruritus, rhinitis, sinusitis, and tearing.
Pregnancy Category   B.

Epinephrine

Brand Name   Epifrin.
Class of Drug   Glaucoma. Adrenergic agonist.
Indications   Primary OAG (POAG).
Dosage Form   Topical ophthalmic solution 0.5%, 1%, 2%.
Dose   1 drop once or two times per day.
Contraindications   Should not be used in patients who have had an attack of
                         NAG since dilation of the pupil may trigger an acute attack.
                         Do not use in patients who are hypersensitive the product or
                         any of its components .
Warnings   Use with caution in patients with hypertensive cardiovascular
                         disease or coronary artery disease. Contains sodium metabi-
                         sulfite, a sulfite that may cause allergic-type reactions inclu-
                         ding anaphylactic symptoms and life-threatening or less-se-
                         vere asthmatic episodes in certain susceptible people. Overall
                         prevalence of sulfite sensitivity in the general population is
                         unknown and probably low; sulfite sensitivity is seen more
                         frequently in asthmatic than in nonasthmatic people.

Adverse Reactions	Include eye pain or ache, brow ache, headache, conjunctival hyperemia, and allergic lid reactions. Adrenochrome deposits in the conjunctiva and cornea after prolonged epinephrine therapy have been reported. Reported to produce reversible macular edema in some aphakic patients.
Pregnancy Category	C.
Drug Interaction	Should be used cautiously in patients with hyperthyroidism, hypertension,heart disease (including coronary insufficiency, angina pectoris, and patients receiving digitalis), cardiac arrhythmias, diabetes, or patients with unstable vasomotor system. All vasopressors should be used cautiously in patients taking MAOIs. Should not be administered concomitantly with other sympathomimetic drugs because of possible additive effects and increased toxicity. Alpha-adrenergic-blocking agents may reduce the vasopressor response to epinephrine by causing vasodilation. Beta-adrenergic-blocking drugs may block the cardiac and bronchodilating effects of epinephrine. Administration of epinephrine to patients receiving anesthesia with cyclopropane or halogenated hydrocarbons, such as halothane, which sensitize the myocardium, may induce cardiac arrhythmia. Should be used cautiously with other drugs (e.g., digitalis glycosides) that sensitize the myocardium to the actions of sympathomimetic agents. Drugs such as reserpine and methyldopa, that reduce the amount of norepinephrine in sympathetic nerve endings, may reduce the pressor response to epinephrine. Diuretic agents also may decrease vascular response to pressor drugs such as epinephrine. May antagonize the neuron blockade produced by guanethidine, resulting in decreased antihypertensive effect and requiring increased dosage of the latter.

Etanercept

Brand Name	Enbrel.
Class of Drug	Binds specifically to TNF and blocks its interaction with cell-surface TNF receptor. TNF is a naturally occurring cytokine that is involved in normal inflammatory and immune responses.
Indications	Rheumatoid arthritis, polyarticular-course JRA, psoriatic arthritis, ankylosing spondylitis, adult patients (18 years or older) with chronic moderate to severe plaque psoriasis who are candidates for systemic therapy or phototherapy.*Off-label*: uveitis and childhood uveitis in association with JRA, Wegener's granulomatosis, and juvenile spondyloarthropathies.

Dosage Form	Powder for subcutaneous injection 25 mg. Powder for reconstitution with 1 ml of sterile bacteriostatic water for subsequent parenteral administration.
Dose	Recommended dose for adult patients with rheumatoid arthritis, psoriatic arthritis, or ankylosing spondylitis is 50 mg per week given as two 25-mg subcutaneous injections at separate sites. Dose should be administered as two 25 mg injections given either on the same day or 3 or 4 days apart. Doses higher than 50 mg per week are not recommended. Recommended starting dose for adult patients with plaque psoriasis is 50 mg given two times per weekly (administered 3 to 4 days apart) for 3 months followed by a reduction to a maintenance dose of 50 mg per week. Recommended dose for pediatric patients ages 4–17 years of age with active polyarticular-course JRA is 0.8 mg/kg per week (up to a maximum of 50 mg per week). The maximum dose that should be administered at a single injection site is 25 mg (1.0 ml).
Contraindications	In patients with sepsis or a known hypersensitivity the product or any of its components.
Warnings	Serious and potentially fatal acute and chronic infections have been described. New onset or exacerbation of preexisting CNS demyelinating disorders. Cases of transverse myelitis, optic neuritis, multiple sclerosis, and new-onset or exacerbation of seizure disorders have been observed. Rare reports of pancytopenia, including aplastic anemia. The potential role of TNF-blocking therapy in the development of malignancies is not known.
Adverse Reactions	Increased risk of serious infections and sepsis. Injection site reactions, including erythema, itching, and swelling. Development of autoantibodies, lupus-like syndrome, anticardiolipin antibodies. Controversial adverse effects and fatality in patients with heart failure. Rule out prior tuberculosis (TB) infection with purified protein derivative (PPD) and chest X-ray (CXR). Monitor CBC with differential, ALT, and AST every 2 weeks for the first month then every 4–6 weeks.
Pregnancy Category	B.
Drug Interactions	Pharmacokinetics was unaltered by concomitant methotrexate in rheumatoid arthritis patients. It is not known whether this drug is excreted in human milk or absorbed systemically after ingestion. Concurrent administration with anakinra (an IL-1 antagonist) has been associated with an increased risk of serious infections, increased risk of neutropenia, and no additional benefit compared with these medicinal products alone.

Etidocaine

Class of Drug	Local anesthetic.
Indications	Local anesthesia.
Dosage Form	Parenteral for injection.
Dose	Maximum 4 mg/kg body weight. Rapid onset; lasts for 4–8 h.
Contraindications	*Most significant*: Adams–Stokes syndrome, lidocaine toxicity, severe heart block. *Significant*: congestive heart failure, hypovolemia, incomplete AV heart block, reduced hepatic blood flow, shock, sinus bradycardia, Wolff–Parkinson–White pattern. *Possibly significant*: renal disease.
Warnings	Local anesthetic solutions containing antimicrobial preservatives (e.g., methylparaben) should not be used for epidural anesthesia because the safety of these agents has not been established with regard to intrathecal injection, either intentional or accidental. Vasopressor agents administered for the treatment of hypotension related to caudal or other epidural blocks should not be used in the presence of ergot-type oxytocic drugs since severe persistent hypertension and even rupture of cerebral blood vessels may occur.
Adverse Reactions	Allergic reactions, anaphylaxis, CNS toxicity, erythema, methemoglobinemia, myocardial dysfunction, nausea, pruritus, skin rash, sneezing, urticaria, vasodilation of blood vessels, vomiting.
Pregnancy Category	B.
Drug Interactions	Possibly safe in pregnancy. It is not known whether this drug or its metabolites are excreted in human milk. *Relative contraindication*: risk of systemic toxicity possible in pediatric patients.

Erythromycin

Brand Name	Ilotycin; Romycin.
Class of Drug	Antibiotic. Suppresses bacterial protein synthesis.
Indications	Superficial ocular infections involving the conjunctiva or cornea caused by organisms susceptible to erythromycin. Prophylaxis of ophthalmia neonatorum caused by *N. gonorrhoeae*. Active against the following organisms: *S. pyogenes* (group A beta-hemolytic streptococci), alpha-hemolytic streptococci (viridans group), *S. aureus* (resistant organisms may emerge during treatment), *S. pneumoniae*, *Mycoplasma pneumoniae*, *Treponema pallidum*, *Corynebacterium diphtheriae*, *Corynebacterium minutissimum*, *Entamoeba histolytica*,

Listeria monocytogenes, N. gonorrhoeae, Bordetella pertussis, Legionella pneumophila (agent of Legionnaires' disease), Ureaplasma urealyticum, C. trachomatis.

Dosage Form Ointment 5 mg/g (0.5%).

Dose Prophylaxis of neonatal gonococcal or chlamydial conjunctivitis: 0.5 cm to 1 cm in length into each conjunctival sac. Conjunctivitis of the newborn caused by C. trachomatis: oral erythromycin suspension 50 mg/kg per day in four divided doses for at least 2 weeks.

Contraindications In patients with a known hypersensitivity to the product or any of its components. Oral erythromycin is contraindicated in patients taking terfenadine, astemizole, or cisapride.

Warnings Oral erythromycin: Reports of hepatic dysfunction, including increased liver enzymes and hepatocellular and/or cholestatic hepatitis with or without jaundice. Reports suggesting erythromycin does not reach the fetus in adequate concentration to prevent congenital syphilis. Infants born to women treated during pregnancy with oral erythromycin for early syphilis should be treated with an appropriate penicillin regimen. Rhabdomyolysis with or without renal impairment has been reported in seriously ill patients receiving erythromycin concomitantly with lovastatin; therefore, patients receiving concomitant lovastatin and erythromycin should be carefully monitored for creatine kinase (CK) and serum transaminase levels.

Pseudomembranous colitis has been reported with nearly all antibacterial agents, including erythromycin, and may range in severity from mild to life threatening; therefore, it is important to consider this diagnosis in patients who present with diarrhea subsequent to the administration of antibacterial agents. Treatment with antibacterial agents alters the normal flora of the colon and may permit overgrowth of clostridia. Studies indicate that a toxin produced by C. difficile is a primary cause of antibiotic-associated colitis. After diagnosis of pseudomembranous colitis has been established, therapeutic measures should be initiated. Mild cases of pseudomembranous colitis usually respond to discontinuation of the drug alone. In moderate to severe cases, consideration should be given to management with fluids and electrolytes, protein supplementation, and treatment with an antibacterial drug clinically effective against C. difficile colitis.

Adverse Reactions Oral erythromycin: Most frequent—gastrointestinal, which are dose-related; they include nausea, vomiting, abdominal pain, diarrhea, and anorexia. Symptoms of hepatitis, hepatic dysfunction and/or abnormal LFT results may occur. Onset of pseudomembranous colitis symptoms may occur during or after antibacterial treatment. Rarely, erythromycin has been associated with the production of ventricular arrhythmias, including ventricular tachycardia and torsades de pointes, in individuals with prolonged QT interval. Allergic reactions ranging from urticaria to anaphylaxis have occurred. Skin reactions ranging from mild eruptions to erythema multiforme, Stevens–Johnson syndrome, and toxic epidermal necrolysis have been reported rarely. There have been isolated reports of reversible hearing loss occurring chiefly in patients with renal insufficiency and in patients receiving high doses of erythromycin. Since erythromycin is principally excreted by the liver, caution should be exercised when administered to patients with impaired hepatic function. There have been reports that erythromycin may aggravate the weakness of patients with myasthenia gravis. Prolonged or repeated use may result in an overgrowth of nonsusceptible bacteria or fungi. If superinfection occurs, erythromycin should be discontinued and appropriate therapy instituted.

Pregnancy Category B.

Drug Interactions *Oral erythromycin*: excreted in human milk; caution should be exercised when administered to a nursing woman. *Drug interactions*: in patients who are receiving high doses of theophylline, may be associated with an increase in serum theophylline levels and potential theophylline toxicity; in case of theophylline toxicity and/or elevated serum theophylline levels, the dose of theophylline should be reduced while the patient is receiving concomitant erythromycin therapy.

Concomitant administration with digoxin has been reported to result in elevated digoxin serum levels. Reports of increased anticoagulant effects when used concomitantly with oral anticoagulants; increased anticoagulation effects due to interactions of erythromycin with oral anticoagulants may be more pronounced in the elderly. Concurrent use with ergotamine or dihydroergotamine has been associated in some patients with acute ergot toxicity characterized by severe peripheral vasospasm and dysesthesia. Reported to decrease the clearance of triazolam and midazolam and, thus, may increase the pharmacologic effect of these benzodiazepines. In patients concurrently taking drugs metabolized by the cytochrome P-450 system, may be associated with elevations in serum levels of these other drugs. Reports of interactions with carbamazepine, cyclosporine, tacrolimus, hexobarbital, phenytoin, alfentanil, cisapride, disopyramide, lovastatin, bromocriptine, valproate, terfenadine, and astemizole. Serum concentrations of drugs metabolized by the cytochrome P-450 system should be monitored closely in patients concurrently receiving erythromycin. Reported to significantly alter the metabolism of the nonsedating antihistamines terfenadine and astemizole when taken concomitantly. Rare cases of serious cardiovascular adverse events, including electrocardiographic QT/QT c interval prolongation, cardiac arrest, *torsades de pointes*, and other ventricular arrhythmias, have been observed. In addition, deaths have been reported rarely with concomitant administration of terfenadine and erythromycin.

Postmarketing reports of drug interactions when erythromycin is coadministered with cisapride, resulting in cardiac arrhythmias (QT prolongation, ventricular tachycardia, ventricular fibrillation, and *torsades de pointes*), most likely due to the inhibition of hepatic metabolism of cisapride by erythromycin. Fatalities have been reported.

Drug/laboratory test interactions: interferes with fluorometric determination of urinary catecholamines.

Famciclovir

Brand Name Famvir.

Class of Drug Antiviral.

Indications Acute herpes zoster (shingles); treatment or suppression of recurrent genital herpes in immunocompetent patients; recurrent mucocutaneous herpes simplex infections in HIV-infected patients.

Dosage Form Oral tablet.

Dose *Herpes zoster infections*: 500 mg every 8 h for 7 days. Therapy should be initiated promptly as soon as herpes zoster is diagnosed. *Herpes simplex infections*: Recurrent genital herpes—125 mg two times per day for 5 days; initiate therapy at the first sign or symptom if medical management of a genital herpes recurrence is indicated. Suppression of recurrent genital herpes—250 mg two times per day for up to 1 year. HIV-infected patients—For recurrent orolabial or genital herpes simplex infection, 500 mg two times per day for 7 days. In patients with reduced renal function or undergoing hemodialysis, dosage reduction is recommended. Famvir may be taken without regard to meals.

Contraindications In patients with a known hypersensitivity to the product or any of its components, and to Denavir (penciclovir cream).

Warnings Dosage adjustment is recommended when administering to patients with CrCl values <60 ml/min. In patients with underlying renal disease who have received inappropriately high doses for their level of renal function, acute renal failure has been reported.

Adverse Reactions *Nervous system*: headache, paresthesia, migraine, hallucinations, and confusion (including delirium, disorientation, confusional state, occurring predominantly in the elderly). *Gastrointestinal*: nausea, vomiting, diarrhea, flatulence, abdominal pain. *Body as a whole*: fatigue. *Skin and appendages*: pruritus, rash, urticaria. *Reproductive female*: dysmenorrhea. *Laboratory abnormalities*: anemia, leukopenia, neutropenia, increase of AST (SGOT), ALT (SGPT), total bilirubin, serum creatinine, amylase, lipase.

Pregnancy Category C.

Drug Interactions Due to the potential for additive or synergistic impairment of renal function, care should be taken when administering Prograf with drugs that may be associated with renal dysfunction. These include, but are not limited to, aminoglycosides, amphotericin B, and cisplatin. Initial clinical experience with the coadministration of Prograf and cyclosporine resulted in additive/synergistic nephrotoxicity. Patients switched from cyclosporine to Prograf should receive the first Prograf dose no sooner than 24 h after the last cyclosporine dose. Dosing may be further delayed in the presence of elevated cyclosporine levels. Since it is metabolized mainly by the CYP3A enzyme systems, substances known to induce or inhibit these enzymes may affect the metabolism or bioavailability of Prograf. Immunosuppressants may affect vaccination.

FK 506

Brand Name	Prograf. Ointment: Protopic.
Class of Drug	Transcription factor inhibitor. T-cell inhibition similar to CSA. Macrolide antibiotic.
Indications	Prophylaxis of organ rejection for patients undergoing allogenic liver transplantation. Also used for prophylaxis of organ rejection in heart, kidney, and small-bowel transplantation. *Other uses*: refractory noninfectious uveitis (e.g. Adamantiades–Behçet disease), psoriasis, nephritic syndrome, *Topical indication*: atopic dermatitis.
Dosage Form	*Oral capsules*: 0.5 mg, 1 mg, 5 mg anhydrous drug. *Solution for IV injection*: 5 mg/ml. *Topical ointment*: 0.03% or 0.1%. *Sterile solution for IV injection*: equivalent of 5 mg anhydrous FK 506 in 1 ml polyoxyl 60 hydrogenated castor oil and dehydrated alcohol; supplied as an ampule, diluted in either 0.9% sodium chloride or 5% dextrose in water before use.
Dose	*Oral dose for refractory noninfectious uveitis*: daily dose of 0.1–0.15 mg/kg per day. Higher doses (0.15 mg and 2.0 mg/kg per day) produce undesirable side effects and require careful monitoring. Trough levels to be maintained between 15 and 25 mg/ml. *IV*: Recommended starting dose 0.03–0.05 mg/kg per day as continuous i.v. infusion. Adult patients should receive doses at the lower end of the dosing range. Concomitant adrenal corticosteroid therapy is recommended early posttransplantation. Continuous i.v. infusion should be continued only until the patient can tolerate oral administration of capsules.
Contraindications	In patients with hypersensitivity to the product or its vehicle.
Warnings	Increased susceptibility to infection and possible development of lymphoma may result from immunosuppression. Because of its extensive metabolism by the liver, blood levels of FK 506 may be significantly increased in patients with hepatic impairment, and patients with underlying renal disease may require dosage adjustment. Elderly patients and patients with diabetes mellitus and systemic hypertension also require vigilant monitoring. Use during pregnancy has been associated with neonatal hyperkalemia and renal dysfunction and should be reserved for circumstances in which potential benefit to mother justifies risk to fetus; avoid during nursing. CSA and FK 506 should not be used simultaneously.

Metabolized by cytochrome P-450; therefore, drugs that either potentiate or inhibit these enzymes produce corresponding changes in FK 506 metabolism. Vaccinations may be less effective during treatment. Live vaccines should be avoided.

Adverse Reactions Nephrotoxicity, systemic hypertension, electrolyte disturbance, hyperglycemia, GI symptoms, opportunistic bacterial, viral and fungal infections, hemolytic anemia.*Neurologic*: headache, dizziness, paresthesias, tremors, sleep disturbances, expressive aphasia, seizures, akinetic mutism, encephalopathy, coma. *Protopic*: no phototoxicity or photoallergenicity detected in clinical studies. Monitor complete hemogram, LFTs, serum BUN, and creatinine before initiation of therapy. Every 3–4 months, repeated CrCl determination, blood pressure.

Pregnancy Category C.

Drug Interactions Has been associated with neonatal hyperkalemia and renal dysfunction during pregnancy and should be reserved for circumstances in which the potential benefit to the mother justifies the risk to the fetus. Should be avoided during nursing. Experience in pediatric kidney transplant patients is limited. Ointment 0.03% may be used in pediatric patients 2 years of age and older. Due to the potential for additive or synergistic impairment of renal function, care should be taken when administering with drugs that may be associated with renal dysfunction. These include, but are not limited to, aminoglycosides, amphotericin B, and cisplatin. Initial clinical experience with the coadministration with CSA resulted in additive/synergistic nephrotoxicity. Patients switched from CSA to FK 506 should receive the first FK 506 dose no sooner than 24 h after the last CSA dose. Dosing may be further delayed in the presence of elevated CSA levels.

Metabolized mainly by the cytochrome P-450 enzyme systems; substances known to inhibit or induce these enzymes may affect the metabolism or the bioavailability of FK 506. Monitoring blood concentrations and appropriate dosage adjustments are essential when such drugs are used concomitantly. *Drugs that may increase blood concentrations* (this list is not all-inclusive): Calcium-channel blockers—diltiazem, nicardipine, nifedipine, verapamil. Antifungal agents—clotrimazole, fluconazole, itraconazole, ketoconazole. Macrolide antibiotics—clarithromycin, erythromycin, troleandomycin. Gastrointestinal prokinetic agents—cisapride, metoclopramide. Other drugs—bromocriptine, cimetidine, cyclosporine, danazol, ethinyl estradiol, methylprednisolone, omeprazole, protease inhibitors, nefazodone. *Drugs that may decrease blood concentrations* (this list is not all inclusive): Anticonvulsants:—carbamazepine, phenobarbital, phenytoin. Antibiotics—rifabutin, rifampin. Herbal preparations—St. John's wort.

Fluconazole

Brand Name Diflucan.

Class of Drug Antifungal.

Indications Vaginal candidiasis (vaginal yeast infections due to *Candida*), oropharyngeal and esophageal candidiasis. In open, non-comparative studies of relatively small numbers of patients, effective for the treatment of *Candida* UTIs, peritonitis, and systemic *Candida* infections, including candidemia, disseminated candidiasis, and pneumonia. Cryptococcal meningitis; studies comparing Diflucan to amphotericin B in non-HIV-infected patients have not been conducted. Prophylaxis to decrease the incidence of candidiasis in patients undergoing bone marrow transplantation who receive cytotoxic chemotherapy and/or radiation therapy.

Dosage Form Oral tablets, oral suspension, injection.

Dose *Vaginal candidiasis*: Single dose, no repeat—150 mg as a single oral dose. Multiple dose—daily dose, same for oral and i.v. administration. In general, a loading dose of twice the daily dose is recommended on the first day of therapy to result in plasma concentrations close to steady-state by the second day of therapy. *Oropharyngeal candidiasis*: 200 mg on the first day, followed by 100 mg once per day; treatment should be continued for at least 2 weeks to decrease the likelihood of relapse. *Esophageal candidiasis*: 200 mg on the first day, followed by 100 mg once per day; doses up to 400 mg/day may be used; patients should be treated for a minimum of 3 weeks and for at least 2 weeks following resolution of symptoms. *Systemic* Candida *infections*: doses up to 400 mg per day have been used. *UTIs and peritonitis*: daily doses of 50–200 mg have been used. *Cryptococcal meningitis*: 400 mg on the first day, followed by 200 mg once per day; 400 mg once per day may be used; initial therapy duration 10–12 weeks after the cerebrospinal fluid becomes culture-negative; for suppression of relapse of cryptococcal meningitis in patients with AIDS, 200 mg once per day. *Prophylaxis in patients undergoing bone marrow transplantation*: 400 mg once per day; patients anticipated to have severe granulocytopenia (less than 500 neutrophils per cubic millimeter) should start Diflucan prophylaxis several days before anticipated onset of neutropenia and continue for 7 days after the neutrophil count rises above 1,000 cells per cubic millimeter.

The following dose equivalency scheme should generally provide equivalent exposure in pediatric and adult patients: pediatric patients 3 mg/kg equivalent to adults 100 mg; pediatric patients 6 mg/kg equivalent to adults 200 mg; pediatric patients 12 mg/kg* equivalent to adults 400 mg. Absolute adult doses exceeding 600 mg/day are not recommended. (*Some older children may have clearances similar to that of adults.)

Contraindications In patients who have shown hypersensitivity to the product or any of its components. There is no information regarding cross-hypersensitivity between fluconazole and other azole antifungal agents. Caution should be used in prescribing to patients with hypersensitivity to other azoles. Coadministration of terfenadine is contraindicated in patients receiving Diflucan (fluconazole) at multiple doses of 400 mg or higher based upon results of a multiple-dose interaction study. Coadministration of cisapride is contraindicated.

Warnings *Hepatic injury*: Has been associated with rare cases of serious hepatic toxicity, including fatalities, primarily in patients with serious underlying medical conditions. The spectrum of these reactions has ranged from mild transient elevations in transaminases to clinical hepatitis, cholestasis, and fulminant hepatic failure, including fatalities. Instances of fatal hepatic reactions were noted to occur primarily in patients with serious underlying medical conditions (predominantly AIDS or malignancy) and often while taking multiple concomitant medications. Transient hepatic reactions, including hepatitis and jaundice, have occurred among patients with no other identifiable risk factors. *Anaphylaxis*: reported in rare cases. *Dermatologic*: Patients have rarely developed exfoliative skin disorders during treatment; patients who develop rashes during treatment should be monitored closely and the drug discontinued if lesions progress.

Precautions: General—some azoles, including fluconazole, have been associated with prolongation of the QT interval on electrocardiogram. During postmarketing surveillance, there have been very rare cases of QT prolongation and torsade de pointes. Should be administered with caution to patients with these potentially proarrhythmic conditions.

Adverse Reactions Headache, nausea, abdominal pain, diarrhea, dyspepsia, dizziness, taste perversion, skin rash, vomiting. Rarely, angioedema and anaphylactic reaction have been reported. The following events have occurred under conditions where a causal association is uncertain: Cardiovascular—QT prolongation, torsade de pointes. CNS—seizures. Dermatologic—exfoliative skin disorders, including Stevens–Johnson syndrome and toxic epidermal necrolysis; alopecia. Hematopoietic and lymphatic—leukopenia, including neutropenia and agranulocytosis; thrombocytopenia. Metabolic—hypercholesterolemia, hypertriglyceridemia, hypokalemia. Adverse reactions in children—most commonly reported events were vomiting, abdominal pain, nausea, diarrhea. The majority of treatment-related laboratory abnormalities were elevations of transaminases or alkaline phosphatase.

Pregnancy Category C.

Flucytosine

Brand Name   Ancobon.
Class of Drug   Antifungal agent.
Indications   Only in the treatment of serious infections caused by suscep-
                          tible strains of*Candida* and/or *Cryptococcus*. *Candida*: septi-
                          cemia, endocarditis, and urinary system infections have been
                          effectively treated. limited trials in pulmonary infections jus-
                          tify use. *Cryptococcus*: meningitis and pulmonary infections
                          have been treated effectively; studies in septicemias and UTIs
                          are limited, but good responses have been reported.
Dosage Form   Capsules for oral administration 250 mg, 500 mg
Dose   Usual dosage is 50–150 mg/kg per day administered in divi-
                          ded doses at 6-h intervals. Nausea or vomiting may be redu-
                          ced or avoided if given a few at a time over a 15-min period. If
                          BUN or serum creatinine is elevated or if there are other signs
                          of renal impairment, initial dose should be at the lower level.
Contraindications   In patients with a known hypersensitivity to the product or
                          any of its components.
Warnings   Must be given with extreme caution to patients with impaired
                          renal function. Since Ancobon is excreted primarily by the
                          kidneys, renal impairment may lead to accumulation of the
                          drug. Blood concentrations should be monitored to determi-
                          ne adequacy of renal excretion in such patients. Dosage ad-
                          justments should be made in patients with renal insufficiency
                          to prevent progressive accumulation of active drug. Must be
                          given with extreme caution to patients with bone marrow de-
                          pression; patients may be more prone to depression of bone
                          marrow function if they: (1) have a hematologic disease, (2)
                          are being treated with radiation or drugs that depress bone
                          marrow, or (3) have a history of treatment with such drugs or
                          radiation. Bone marrow toxicity can be irreversible and may
                          lead to death in immunosuppressed patients. Frequent mo-
                          nitoring of hepatic function and the hematopoietic system is
                          indicated during therapy. Before therapy is instituted, elec-
                          trolytes (because of hypokalemia) and hematologic and renal
                          status should be determined. Blood concentrations, kidney
                          function, hematologic status (leucocyte and thrombocyte
                          count), and liver function (alkaline phosphatase, SGOT, and
                          SGPT) should be determined at frequent intervals during
                          treatment, as indicated.
Adverse Reactions   *Cardiovascular*: cardiac arrest, myocardial toxicity, ventricular
                          dysfunction. *Respiratory*: respiratory arrest, chest pain, dys-
                          pnea. *Dermatologic*: rash, pruritus, urticaria, photosensitivity.
                          Gastrointestinal: nausea, emesis, abdominal pain, diarrhea,
                          anorexia, dry mouth, duodenal ulcer, gastrointestinal hemor-
                          rhage, acute hepatic injury with possible fatal outcome in

debilitated patients, hepatic dysfunction, jaundice, ulcerative colitis, bilirubin elevation. *Genitourinary*: azotemia, creatinine and BUN elevation, crystalluria, renal failure. *Hematologic*: anemia, agranulocytosis, aplastic anemia, eosinophilia, leukopenia, pancytopenia, thrombocytopenia. *Neurologic*: ataxia, hearing loss, headache, paresthesia, Parkinsonism, peripheral neuropathy, pyrexia, vertigo, sedation, convulsions. *Psychiatric*: confusion, hallucinations, psychosis. *Miscellaneous*: fatigue, hypoglycemia, hypokalemia, weakness, allergic reactions, Lyell's syndrome.

Pregnancy Category C.

Drug Interactions Cytosine arabinoside, a cytostatic agent, has been reported to inactivate antifungal activity by competitive inhibition. Drugs that impair glomerular filtration may prolong the biological half-life of flucytosine. Antifungal synergism between Ancobon and polyene antibiotics, particularly amphotericin B, has been reported.*Drug/laboratory test interactions*: measurement of serum creatinine levels should be determined by the Jaffe method since Ancobon does not interfere with the determination of creatinine values by this method, as it does when the dry-slide enzymatic method with the Kodak Ektachem analyzer is used.

Fluorescein Sodium

Brand Name Fluorescite Injection.

Class of Drug Diagnostic aid.

Indications Diagnostic fluorescein angiography or angioscopy of the fundus and iris vasculature.

Dosage Form Ampule: 10% in 5-ml ampule, 25% in 2-ml ampule.

Dose Parenteral drug products should be inspected visually for particulate matter and discoloration prior to administration whenever solution and container permit. Do not mix or dilute with other solutions or drugs. A syringe filled with fluorescein is attached to transparent tubing and a 25-gauge scalp-vein needle for injection. Insert the needle and draw the patient's blood to the hub of the syringe so that a small air bubble separates the patient's blood in the tubing from the fluorescein. With the room lights on, slowly inject the blood back into the vein while watching the skin over the needle tip. If the needle has extravasated, the patient's blood will be seen to bulge the skin, and the injection should be stopped before any fluorescein is injected. When assured that extravasation has not occurred, the room light may be turned off and the fluorescein injection completed. Luminescence appears in the retina and choroidal vessels in 9–14 s and can be observed by standard viewing equipment. If potential allergy is suspected, an intradermal skin test may be performed prior to i.v. administration, i.e., 0.05 ml injected intradermally to be evaluated 30–60 min following injection. For children, the dose is calculated on the basis of 35 mg for each 10 lb body weight.

Contraindications In patients who have shown hypersensitivity to the product or any of its components.

Warnings *Not for intrathecal use; for ophthalmic use only.* Care must be taken to avoid extravasation during injection as the high pH of fluorescein solution can result in severe local tissue damage. The following complications resulting from extravasation have been noted: sloughing of the skin, superficial phlebitis, subcutaneous granuloma, and toxic neuritis along the median curve in the antecubital area. Complications resulting from extravasation can cause severe pain in the arm for up to several hours. When significant extravasation occurs, the injection should be discontinued and conservative measures to treat damaged tissue and relieve pain should be implemented. Do not mix or dilute with other solutions or drugs in syringe. Flush i.v. cannulas before and after drugs are injected to avoid physical incompatibility reactions. Rare cases of death due to anaphylaxis have been reported. Caution is to be exercised in patients with a history of allergy or bronchial asthma. An emergency tray including such items as 0.1% epinephrine for i.v. or i.m. use; an antihistamine, soluble steroid, and aminophylline for i.v. use; and oxygen should always be available in the event of possible reaction to fluorescein injection.

Adverse Reactions Nausea and headache, gastrointestinal distress, syncope, vomiting, and hypotension and other symptoms and signs of hypersensitivity have occurred. Cardiac arrest, basilar artery ischemia, severe shock, convulsions, thrombophlebitis at the injection site, and rare cases of death have been reported. Extravasation of the solution at the injection site causes intense pain at the site and a dull aching pain in the injected arm. Generalized hives and itching, bronchospasm, and anaphylaxis have been reported. A strong taste may develop after injection.*Information for patients*: Skin will attain a temporary yellowish discoloration. Urine attains a bright yellow color. Discoloration of the skin fades in 6–12 h and urine fluorescein dissipates in 24–36 h.

Drug Interactions *Avoid* angiography on patients who are pregnant, especially those in the first trimester. There have been no reports of fetal complications from injection during pregnancy. Has been demonstrated to be excreted in human milk; caution should be exercised when administered to a nursing woman.

Brand Name Fluor-I-Strip A.T. 1 mg; Fluor-I-Strip 9 mg.
Class of Drug Diagnostic aid.

Indications   For staining the anterior segment of the eye when: (a) delineating a corneal injury, herpetic lesion, or foreign body; (b) determining the site of an intraocular injury; (c) fitting contact lenses; (d) testing to ascertain postoperative closure of the sclerocorneal wound in delayed anterior chamber reformation; (e) testing lacrimal drainage.

Dosage Form   Fluorescein sodium 1 mg, 9 mg per strip.

Dose   Gently touch the strip to the inferior fornix.

Warnings   Never use while the patient is wearing soft contact lenses because the lenses may become stained. Whenever fluorescein is used, flush the eyes with sterile, normal saline solution, and wait at least 1 h before replacing the lenses.

Fluorescein Sodium and Benoxinate HCl

Brand Name   Fluress; Flurox; Flurate.

Class of Drug   Diagnostic aid, topical anesthetic.

Indications   For procedures in which a topical ophthalmic anesthetic agent in conjunction with a disclosing agent are indicated: corneal anesthesia of short duration, e.g., tonometry, gonioscopy, removal of corneal foreign bodies, and short corneal and conjunctival procedures.

Dosage Form   Fluorescein sodium 0.25% and benoxinate HCl 0.4%.

Dose   *Usual dosage (removal of foreign bodies and sutures, and for tonometry)*: 1–2 drops (in single installations) in each eye before operating. *Deep ophthalmic anesthesia*: 2 drops in eye(s) at 90-s intervals for three instillations.

Contraindications   In patients with known hypersensitivity to the product or any of its components.

Warnings   Prolonged use of a topical ocular anesthetic is not recommended. It may produce permanent corneal opacification with accompanying visual loss.

Adverse Reactions   *Occasional*: temporary stinging, burning, conjunctival redness. *Rare*: severe, immediate-type, apparently hyperallergic corneal reaction with acute, intense, and diffuse epithelial keratitis, a gray, ground-glass appearance, sloughing or large areas of necrotic epithelium, corneal filaments, and sometimes, iritis with descemetitis.

Pregnancy Category   C.

Fluorometholone

Brand Name	FML; Fluor-Op; Eflone; Flarex; FML Forte; FML S.O.P.
Class of Drug	Topical corticosteroid.
Indications	For the treatment of steroid-responsive inflammation of the palpebral and bulbar conjunctiva, cornea, and anterior segment of the globe.
Dosage Form	Ophthalmic suspension 0.1% (FML, Fluor-Op, Eflone, Flarex). Ophthalmic suspension 0.25% (FML Forte). Ophthalmic ointment 0.1% (FML S.O.P).
Dose	*Suspension*: 1–2 drops four times per day *Ointment*: 1-cm (approx. ½-in.) ribbon applied to the conjunctival sac one to three times per day. During a 24–48 h interval, frequency of dosing may be increased to one application every 4 h. Care should be taken not to discontinue therapy prematurely.
Contraindications	In most viral diseases of the cornea and conjunctiva, including epithelial herpes simplex keratitis (dendritic keratitis), vaccinia, and varicella; mycobacterial infection of the eye; fungal diseases of ocular structures; in patients with a known or suspected hypersensitivity to the product or any of its components or to other corticosteroids.
Warnings	Prolonged use of corticosteroids may result in glaucoma with damage to the optic nerve, defects in visual acuity and fields of vision, and in posterior subcapsular cataract formation. Prolonged use may also suppress the host immune response and thus increase the hazard of secondary ocular infections. Various ocular diseases and long-term use of topical corticosteroids have been known to cause corneal and scleral thinning. Use of topical corticosteroids in the presence of thin corneal or scleral tissue may lead to perforation. Acute purulent infections of the eye may be masked or activity enhanced by the presence of corticosteroid medication. If this product is used for 10 days or longer, IOP should be routinely monitored even though it may be difficult in children and uncooperative patients. Steroids should be used with caution in the presence of glaucoma. IOP should be checked frequently. The use of steroids after cataract surgery may delay healing and increase the incidence of bleb formation.
Adverse Reactions	Include, in decreasing order of frequency, elevation of IOP with possible development of glaucoma and infrequent optic nerve damage, posterior subcapsular cataract formation, delayed wound healing. Although systemic effects are extremely uncommon, there have been rare occurrences of systemic hypercorticoidism after use of topical steroids. Corticosteroid-containing preparations have also been reported to cause acute anterior uveitis and perforation of the globe.

Keratitis, conjunctivitis, corneal ulcers, mydriasis, conjunctival hyperemia, loss of accommodation, and ptosis have occasionally been reported following local use of corticosteroids. Development of secondary ocular infection (bacterial, fungal, viral) has occurred. Fungal and viral infections of the cornea are particularly prone to develop coincidentally with long-term applications of steroids. The possibility of fungal invasion should be considered in any persistent corneal ulceration where steroid treatment has been used. Use of ocular steroids may prolong the course and may exacerbate the severity of many viral infections of the eye (including herpes simplex). Employment of corticosteroid medication in the treatment of patients with a history of herpes simplex requires great caution; frequent slit lamp microscopy is recommended. Corticosteroids are not effective in mustard gas keratitis and Sjögren's keratoconjunctivitis.

Pregnancy Category C.

Brand Name FML-S.

Class of Drug Topical steroid antibiotic.

Indications For steroid-responsive inflammatory ocular conditions for which a corticosteroid is indicated and where superficial bacterial ocular infection or a risk of bacterial ocular infection exists. The use of a combination drug with an anti-infective component is indicated where the risk of superficial ocular infection is high or where there is an expectation that potentially dangerous numbers of bacteria will be present in the eye. The anti-infective drug in this product, sulfacetamide, is active against the following common bacterial eye pathogens:*E. coli, S. aureus, S. pneumoniae, Streptococcus* (viridans group), *H. influenzae, Klebsiella* spp., and *Enterobacter* spp. The product does not provide adequate coverage against *Neisseria* spp. and *S. marcescens*. A significant percentage of staphylococcal isolates are completely resistant to sulfa drugs.

Dosage Form Ophthalmic suspension: fluorometholone 0.1% and sulfacetamide sodium 10%.

Dose 1 drop into the conjunctival sac four times per day. If signs and symptoms fail to improve after 2 days, the patient should be re-evaluated. Dosing may be reduced, but care should be taken not to discontinue therapy prematurely. In chronic conditions, withdrawal of treatment should be carried out by gradually decreasing the frequency of applications.

Contraindications In most viral diseases of the cornea and conjunctiva, including epithelial herpes simplex keratitis (dendritic keratitis), vaccinia, and varicella; mycobacterial infection of the eye; fungal diseases of ocular structures; in patients with a known or suspected hypersensitivity to the product or any of its components, sulfonamides, or other corticosteroids.

Warnings See »FML; Fluor-Op; Eflone; Flarex; FML Forte; FML S.O.P.« *Fatalities have occurred, although rarely, due to severe reactions* to sulfonamides including Stevens–Johnson syndrome, toxic epidermal necrolysis, fulminant hepatic necrosis, agranulocytosis, aplastic anemia, and other blood dyscrasias. Sensitizations may recur when a sulfonamide is readministered, irrespective of the route of administration. If signs of hypersensitivity or other serious reactions occur, discontinue use. Cross-sensitivity among corticosteroids has been demonstrated. A significant percentage of staphylococcal isolates are completely resistant to sulfa drugs.

Adverse Reactions   See »FML; Fluor-Op; Eflone; Flarex; FML Forte; FML S.O.P.« Reactions occurring most often from the presence of the anti-infective ingredient are allergic sensitizations. Fatalities have occurred, although rarely, due to severe reactions to sulfonamides, including Stevens-Johnson syndrome, toxic epidermal necrolysis, fulminant hepatic necrosis, agranulocytosis, aplastic anemia, and other blood dyscrasias. Sulfacetamide sodium may cause local irritation.

Secondary Infection: Has occurred after use of combinations containing corticosteroids and antimicrobials. Fungal infections of the cornea are particularly prone to develop coincidentally with long-term application of corticosteroids. When signs of chronic ocular inflammation persist following prolonged corticosteroid dosing, the possibility of fungal infections of the cornea should be considered. Secondary bacterial ocular infection following suppression of host responses also occurs.

Pregnancy Category   C.
Drug Interactions   Sulfacetamide preparations are incompatible with silver preparations.

5-Fluorouracil (5-FU)

Brand Name   Adrucil.
Class of Drug   Antineoplastic antimetabolite.
Indications   Palliative management of carcinoma of the colon, rectum, breast, stomach, and pancreas. Off-label: adjuvant in glaucoma surgery.
Dosage Form   Single-use vials contain 500 mg of 5-FU in 10 ml.
Dose   Off-label: Intraoperatively in glaucoma surgery: apply a piece of Weck-cell sponge (soaked with 50 mg/cc 5-FU) under the conjunctiva and Tenon's capsule on the sclera of the site of glaucoma surgery. Postoperative subconjunctival injection: 5–10 mg [may be diluted with balanced salt solution (BSS)] injected subconjunctivally intermediately after glaucoma surgery and can be repeated the first 1–2 weeks after surgery.

Contraindications	As cancer chemotherapy: Injection therapy for patients in poor nutritional state, those with depressed bone marrow function, those with potentially serious infections, or in patients with a known hypersensitivity to the product or any of its components.
Warnings	As cancer chemotherapy: daily dose of injection not to exceed 80 mg. It is recommended that patients be hospitalized during their first course of treatment. Should be used with extreme caution in poor-risk patients with a history of high-dose pelvic irradiation or previous use of alkylating agents, those who have a widespread involvement of bone marrow by metastatic tumors, or those with impaired hepatic or renal function. Rarely, unexpected, severe toxicity (e.g., stomatitis, diarrhea, neutropenia, neurotoxicity) associated has been attributed to deficiency of dipyrimidine dehydrogenase activity.
Adverse Reactions	*As cancer chemotherapy*: Patients should be informed of expected toxic effects, particularly oral manifestations; alerted to the possibility of alopecia as a result of therapy; and informed that it is usually a transient effect. A highly toxic drug with a narrow margin of safety. Sever hematological toxicity, gastrointestinal hemorrhage, and even death may result, despite meticulous selection of patients and careful adjustment of dosage. Therapy is to be discontinued promptly whenever one of the following signs of toxicity appears: stomatitis or esophagopharyngitis, leukopenia, or rapid falling WBC, intractable vomiting, diarrhea, gastrointestinal ulceration and bleeding, thrombocytopenia, and hemorrhage from any site. *Off-label*: as an adjuvant in glaucoma surgery: bleb leakage, hypotony, flat anterior chamber, blebitis, endophthalmitis, ocular inflammation, uveitis, epithelial defect, ocular discomfort, decrease of vision; late bleb leak or endophthalmitis may be associated with use for glaucoma surgery.
Pregnancy Category	D.
Drug Interactions	May cause fetal harm when administered to a pregnant woman. Women of childbearing potential should be advised to avoid becoming pregnant while taking the drug and should be told of potential hazard to the fetus. Should be used during pregnancy only if the potential benefit justifies the potential risk to the fetus. Leucovorin calcium may enhance toxicity.

Flurbiprofen

Brand Name	Ocufen.
Class of Drug	NSAID.
Indications	Inhibition of intraoperative miosis.
Dosage Form	Topical ophthalmic solution 0.03%.
Dose	A total of 4 drops administered by instilling 1 drop approximately every half hour beginning 2 h before surgery.
Contraindications	In patients hypersensitive to the product or any of its components .
Warnings	With NSAIDs, there exists the potential for increased bleeding due to interference with thrombocyte aggregation. There have been reports that it may cause increased bleeding of ocular tissues, including hyphemas in conjunction with ocular surgery. Potential for cross-sensitivity to acetylsalicylic acid and other NSAIDs; therefore, caution should be used when treating individuals who have previously exhibited sensitivities to these drugs.
Adverse Reactions	*Precautions*: Wound healing may be delayed with use. It is recommended that the solution be used with caution in surgical patients with known bleeding tendencies or who are receiving other medications that may prolong bleeding time. *Other adverse reactions reported include*: transient burning and stinging and other minor symptoms of ocular irritation, fibrosis, miosis, and mydriasis; increased bleeding tendency of ocular tissues in conjunction with ocular surgery.
Pregnancy Category	C.
Drug Interactions	Although clinical studies with acetylcholine chloride and animal studies with acetylcholine chloride or carbachol revealed no interference, and there is no known pharmacological basis for an interaction, there have been reports that acetylcholine chloride and carbachol have been ineffective when used in patients treated with Ocufen ophthalmic solution.

Fomivirsen Sodium

Brand Name	Vitravene.
Class of Drug	Antiviral.
Indications	For the local treatment of CMV retinitis (CMVR) in patients with AIDS who are intolerant of or have a contraindication to other treatment(s) for CMV retinitis or who were insufficiently responsive to previous treatment(s) for CMV retinitis.

Dosage Form Single-use vials contain 0.25 ml, 6.6 mg/ml.

Dose Treatment involves an induction and a maintenance phase. Recommended dose is 330 µg (0.05 ml). *Induction dose*: one injection every other week for two doses. *Subsequent maintenance doses*: once every 4 weeks after induction. For unacceptable inflammation in the face of controlled CMVR, it is worthwhile interrupting therapy until the level of inflammation decreases and therapy can resume. For patients whose disease progresses during maintenance, an attempt at reinduction at the same dose may result in resumed disease control. *Instructions for intravitreal injection*: administer 0.05 ml/eye to affected eye(s) following application of standard topical and/or local anesthetics and antimicrobials using a 30-gauge needle on a low-volume (e.g., tuberculin) syringe.

Contraindications In patients who have known hypersensitivity to the product or any of its components.

Warnings For intravitreal injection use only. CMVR may be associated with CMV disease elsewhere in the body. Provides localized therapy limited to the treated eye; does not provide treatment for systemic CMV disease. Patients should be monitored for extraocular CMV disease or disease in the contralateral eye. Not recommended for use in patients who have recently (2–4 weeks) been treated with either i.v. or intravitreal cidofovir because of risk of exaggerated ocular inflammation.

Adverse Reactions *Most frequent*: Ocular inflammation (uveitis), including iritis and vitreitis, has been reported to occur in approximately one in four patients. Inflammatory reactions are more common during induction dosing. Delaying additional treatment and the use of topical corticosteroids have been useful in the medical management of inflammatory changes, and with both medical management and time, patients may be able to continue to receive intravitreal injections after the inflammation has resolved. Increased IOP has been commonly reported; the increase is usually a transient event and in most cases, pressure returns to the normal range without any treatment or with temporary use of topical medications. IOP should be monitored at each visit, and elevations of IOP, if sustained, should be managed with medications to lower IOP. *Reported by 5–20% of patients*: Ocular—abnormal vision, anterior chamber inflammation, blurred vision, cataract, conjunctival hemorrhage, decreased visual acuity, desaturation of color vision, eye pain, floaters, increased IOP, photophobia, retinal detachment, retinal edema, retinal hemorrhage, retinal pigment changes, uveitis, vitreitis. Systemic—abdominal pain, anemia, asthenia, diarrhea, fever, headache, infection, nausea, pneumonia, rash, sepsis, sinusitis, systemic CMV, vomiting. *Reported by 2–5% of patients*: Ocular—application-site reaction, conjunctival hyperemia, conjunctivitis, corneal edema, decreased peripheral vision, eye irritation, hypotony, keratic precipitates, optic neuritis, photopsia, retinal vascular disease, visual field defect, vitreous hemorrhage, vitreous opacity. Systemic—abnormal liver function, abnormal thinking, allergic reactions, anorexia, back pain, bronchitis, cachexia, catheter infection, chest pain, decreased weight, dehydration, depression, dizziness, dyspnea, flu syndrome, increased cough, increased gamma-glutamyl transpeptidase (GGTP), kidney failure, lymphoma-like reaction, neuropathy, neutropenia, oral moniliasis, pain, pancreatitis, sweating, thrombocytopenia.

Pregnancy Category   C.
Drug Interactions   Interaction with other drugs in humans has not been studied. Results from in vitro tests demonstrated no inhibition of antihuman cytomegalovirus (HCMV) activity of fomivirsen by AZT or ddC.

Foscarnet Sodium

Brand Name   Foscavir.
Class of Drug   Antiviral.
Indications   *CMVR*: In patients with AIDS. Combination therapy with ganciclovir is indicated for patients who have relapsed after monotherapy with either drug. <u>Safety and efficacy have not been established for treatment of other CMV infections (e.g., pneumonitis, gastroenteritis), congenital or neonatal CMV disease, or nonimmunocompromised individuals.</u> *Acyclovir-resistant mucocutaneous HSV infections*: In immunocompromised patients. *Safety and efficacy have not been established for treatment of other HSV infections (e.g., retinitis, encephalitis), congenital or neonatal HSV disease, or HSV in nonimmunocompromised individuals.*

Dosage Form   Injectable.
Dose   *CMVR*: Induction dose—either 90 mg/kg (1½- to 2-h infusion) every 12 h, or 60 mg/kg (minimum 1-h infusion) every 8 h over 2–3 weeks, depending on clinical response. Maintenance dose—90 mg/kg per day to 120 mg/kg per day (individualized for renal function) given as an i.v. infusion over 2 h. Escalation to 120 mg/kg per day may be considered should early reinduction be required because of retinitis progression. Patients who experience progression of retinitis while receiving maintenance therapy may be re-treated with the induction and maintenance regimens given above or with a combination of Foscavir and ganciclovir. *Acyclovir-resistant HSV*: 40 mg/kg (minimum 1-h infusion) either every 8 or 12 h for 2–3 weeks or until healed. Renal function must be monitored carefully at baseline and during induction and mainte-

nance therapy with appropriate dose adjustments. To reduce the risk of nephrotoxicity, CrCl (milliliters per minute per kilogram) should be calculated even if serum creatinine is within the normal range, and doses should be adjusted accordingly. Because of physical incompatibility, Foscavir and ganciclovir must *not* be mixed.

Contraindications

In patients with clinically significant hypersensitivity to the product or any of its components. During therapy, if CrCl falls below the limits of the dosing nomograms (0.4 ml/min per kilogram), Foscavir should be discontinued and the patient hydrated and monitored daily until resolution of renal impairment is ensured.

Warnings

Renal impairment: The major toxicity is renal impairment, which most likely becomes clinically evident during the second week of induction therapy but may occur at any time during treatment. Renal function should be monitored carefully during both induction and maintenance therapy. *Mineral and electrolyte abnormalities*: Patients should be advised to report symptoms of low ionized calcium such as perioral tingling, numbness in the extremities, and paresthesias. Physicians should be prepared to treat these abnormalities and their sequelae, such as tetany, seizures, or cardiac disturbances. An infusion pump must be used for administration to prevent rapid i.v. infusion. Slowing the infusion rate may decrease or prevent symptoms. *Seizures*: related to mineral and electrolyte abnormalities have been associated with Foscavir treatment. Risk factors associated with seizures included impaired baseline renal function, low total serum calcium, and underlying CNS conditions.

Adverse Reactions

Renal impairment. Mineral and electrolyte abnormalities—has been associated with changes in serum electrolytes, including hypocalcemia, hypophosphatemia, hyperphosphatemia, hypomagnesemia, and hypokalemia; may also be associated with a dose-related decrease in ionized serum calcium, which may not be reflected in total serum calcium. Seizures. Hemopoietic system—anemia, granulocytopenia, neutropenia.

Pregnancy Category

C.

Drug Interactions

Concomitant treatment with i.v. pentamidine may have caused hypocalcemia; one patient died with severe hypocalcemia. Because of tendency to cause renal impairment, should be avoided in combination with potentially nephrotoxic drugs, such as aminoglycosides, amphotericin B, and i.v. pentamidine unless the potential benefits outweigh the risks to the patient. Abnormal renal function has been observed in clinical practice during concomitant use with ritonavir or with ritonavir and saquinavir. Since foscarnet decreases serum concentrations of ionized calcium, concurrent treatment with other drugs known to influence serum calcium concentrations should be used with particular caution.

Ganciclovir Sodium

Brand Name	Vitrasert (implantable); Cytovene.
Class of Drug	Antiviral.
Indications	Prevention of CMV disease in solid organ transplant recipients and in individuals with advanced HIV infection at risk for developing CMV disease. Alternative to i.v. formulation for maintenance treatment of CMV retinitis in immunocompromised patients, including patients with AIDS, in whom retinitis is stable following appropriate induction therapy and for whom the risk of more rapid progression is balanced by the benefit associated with avoiding daily i.v. infusions.
Dosage Form	Oral, injectable, implantable.
Dose	*CMV retinitis*: Induction treatment—5 mg/kg (given i.v. at a constant rate over 1 h) every 12 h for 14–21 days; cytovene capsules should not be used for induction treatment. Maintenance treatment—Cytovene i.v. solution 5 mg/kg given as a constant-rate i.v. infusion over 1 h once per day 7 days per week or 6 mg/kg once per day 5 days per week; or Cytovene capsules 1,000 mg three times per day with food. Alternatively, the dosing regimen of 500 mg six times per day every 3 h with food during waking hours may be used. For patients who experience progression of CMV retinitis while receiving maintenance treatment with either formulation of ganciclovir, reinduction treatment is recommended. *Prevention of CMV disease in patients with advanced HIV infection*: Cytovene capsules 1,000 mg three times per day with food. *Prevention of CMV disease in transplant recipients*: Cytovene i.v. solution 5 mg/kg (given at a constant rate over 1 h) every 12 h for 7–14 days, followed by 5 mg/kg once per day 7 days per week or 6 mg/kg once per day 5 days per week; or Cytovene capsules 1,000 mg three times per day with food. Duration of treatment with solution and capsules in transplant recipients is dependent upon the duration and degree of immunosuppression. CBC, platelet count, and serum creatinine or CrCl values should be followed carefully to allow for dosage adjustments.
Contraindications	In patients with hypersensitivity to the product or any of its components or to acyclovir. Should not be administered if absolute neutrophil count is less than 500 cells/µl or platelet count is less than 25,000 cells/µl. Should, therefore, be used with caution in patients with preexisting cytopenias or with a history of cytopenic reactions to other drugs, chemicals, or irradiation.
Warnings	*Teratogenesis*: Because of the mutagenic and teratogenic potential of ganciclovir, women of childbearing potential should be advised to use effective contraception during treatment. Similarly, men should be advised to practice barrier contraception during and for at least 90 days following treatment. <u>Do not administer i.v. solution by rapid or</u>

bolus i.v. injection; toxicity may be increased as a result of excessive plasma levels; i.m. or subcutaneous injection of reconstituted Cytovene i.v. solution may result in severe tissue irritation due to high pH (11); recommended dose for Cytovene i.v. solution and capsules should not be exceeded; recommended infusion rate for Cytovene i.v. solution should not be exceeded.

Adverse Reactions

Body as a whole: fever, chills, infection, sepsis. *Digestive system*: diarrhea, anorexia, vomiting. *Hematologic*: severe leukopenia, neutropenia, anemia, thrombocytopenia, pancytopenia, bone marrow depression, aplastic anemia. *Nervous system*: neuropathy. *Other*: sweating, pruritus. *Catheter related*: catheter infection, sepsis. *Laboratory abnormalities*: granulocytopenia, anemia, thrombocytopenia, neutropenia, increase of serum creatinine. *Fertility*: it is considered probable that ganciclovir at the recommended doses causes temporary or permanent inhibition of spermatogenesis; animal data also indicate that suppression of fertility in females may occur.

Pregnancy Category

C.

Drug Interactions

A decrease in steady-state ganciclovir AUC observed when didanosine was administered 2 h prior to administration of ganciclovir, but ganciclovir AUC was not affected by the presence of didanosine when the two drugs were administered simultaneously. Mean steady-state ganciclovir AUC decreased in the presence of zidovudine. Since both zidovudine and ganciclovir have the potential to cause neutropenia and anemia, some patients may not tolerate concomitant therapy at full dosage. Ganciclovir AUC increased in the presence of probenecid, Generalized seizures have been reported in patients who received ganciclovir and imipenem-cilastatin. These drugs should not be used concomitantly unless the potential benefits outweigh the risks.

Gatifloxacin

Brand Name

Zymar.

Class of Drug

Fluoroquinolone, antibacterial. Inhibition of DNA gyrase and topoisomerase IV.

Indications

For the treatment of bacterial conjunctivitis caused by susceptible strains of the following organisms: Aerobic gram-positive bacteria—*Corynebacterium propinquum**, *S. aureus*, *S. epidermidis*, *Streptococcus mitis**, *S. pneumoniae*. Aerobic gram-negative bacteria—*H. influenzae*. (*Efficacy for this organism was studied in fewer than ten infections.)

Dosage Form Topical ophthalmic solution 0.3%.

Dose *Bacterial conjunctivitis*: days 1 and 2, 1 drop every 2 h to affected eye(s) while awake up to eight times per day; days 3–7, 1 drop up to four times per day while awake.

Contraindications In patients with a history of hypersensitivity to the product or any of its components or to other quinolones.

Warnings Should not be injected subconjunctivally nor introduced directly into the anterior chamber of the eye. In patients receiving systemic quinolones, including gatifloxacin, serious and occasionally fatal hypersensitivity (anaphylactic) reactions, some following the first dose, have been reported. Some reactions were accompanied by cardiovascular collapse, loss of consciousness, angioedema (including laryngeal, pharyngeal, or facial edema), airway obstruction, dyspnea, urticaria, and itching. If an allergic reaction occurs, discontinue the drug. Serious acute hypersensitivity reactions may require immediate emergency treatment. Oxygen and airway management should be administered as clinically indicated.

Adverse Reactions *Ophthalmic use*: Most frequently reported in the overall study population—conjunctival irritation, increased lacrimation—keratitis, and papillary conjunctivitis (approximately 5–10% of patients). Other reported reactions—chemosis, conjunctival hemorrhage, dry eye, eye discharge, eye irritation, eye pain, eyelid edema, headache, red eye, reduced visual acuity, and taste disturbance (occurring in 1–4% of patients).

Pregnancy Category C.

Drug Interactions Specific drug interaction studies have not been conducted. However, systemic administration of some quinolones has been shown to elevate plasma concentrations of theophylline, interfere with metabolism of caffeine, enhance effects of the oral anticoagulant warfarin and its derivatives, and has been associated with transient elevations in serum creatinine in patients receiving systemic cyclosporine concomitantly.

Gentamicin Sulfate

Brand Name Genoptic; Gentak; Gentacidin.

Class of Drug Antibacterial, aminoglycoside. Inhibits bacterial protein synthesis.

Indications *Gentamicin ophthalmic solution* is indicated in the topical treatment of ocular bacterial infections, including conjunctivitis, keratitis, keratoconjunctivitis, corneal ulcers, blepharitis, blepharoconjunctivitis, acute meibomianitis, and dacryocystitis caused by susceptible strains of S. aureus, S. epidermidis, S. pyogenes, S. pneumoniae, E. aerogenes, E. coli, H. influenzae, K. pneumoniae, N. gonorrhoeae, P. aeruginosa, and S. marcescens.

Dosage Form   Solution: 0.3%. Ointment: 0.3%.

Dose   Solution: 1–2 drops to affected eye(s) every four h. In severe infections, dosage may be increased to as much as 2 drops every hour. Ointment: small amount [1-cm (approx. ½-in.) ribbon] to affected eye(s) two to three times per day.

Contraindications   In patients with a known hypersensitivity to the product or any of its components.

Warnings   <u>Ointment and solution are not for injection</u>. They should never be injected subconjunctivally nor should they be directly introduced into the anterior chamber of the eye.

Adverse Reactions   Prolonged use of topical antibiotics may give rise to overgrowth of nonsusceptible organisms, including fungi. Bacterial resistance to gentamicin may also develop. Bacterial and fungal corneal ulcers have developed during treatment with gentamicin ophthalmic preparations.Most frequent: ocular burning and irritation upon drug instillation, nonspecific conjunctivitis, conjunctival epithelial defects, and conjunctival hyperemia. Others: rarely—allergic reactions, thrombocytopenic purpura, hallucinations.

Pregnancy Category   C.

Drug Interactions   No published carcinogenicity or impairment of fertility studies on gentamicin. Aminoglycoside antibiotics have been found to be nonmutagenic.

Brand Name   Pred-G.

Class of Drug   Topical anti-inflammatory, antibacterial.

Indications   Suspension is indicated for steroid-responsive inflammatory ocular conditions for which a corticosteroid is indicated and where superficial bacterial ocular infection or a risk of bacterial ocular infection exists. Ocular steroids are indicated in inflammatory conditions of the palpebral and bulbar conjunctiva, cornea, and anterior segment of the globe where the inherent risk of steroid use in certain infective conjunctivitides is accepted in order to obtain a diminution in edema and inflammation. Also indicated in chronic anterior uveitis, and corneal injury from chemical, radiation, or thermal burns or penetration of foreign bodies. The particular anti-infective drug in this product is active against the following common bacterial eye pathogens:S. aureus, S. pyogenes, S. pneumoniae, E. aerogenes, E. coli, H. influenzae, K. pneumoniae, N. gonorrhoeae, P. aeruginosa, and S. marcescens.

Dosage Form   Ophthalmic suspension: gentamicin 0.3%; prednisolone acetate 1%. Ophthalmic ointment: gentamicin 0.3%; prednisolone acetate 0.6%.

Dose   Solution: 1 drop into the conjunctival sac two to four times per day. During the initial 24–48 h, dosing frequency may be increased, if necessary, up to 1 drop every hour. Care should be taken not to discontinue therapy prematurely. If signs and symptoms fail to improve after 2 days, the patient should be re-evaluated. *Ointment*: a small amount [1-cm (approx. ½-in.) ribbon] applied in the conjunctival sac one to three times per day. Care should be taken not to discontinue therapy prematurely.

Contraindications

In most viral diseases of the cornea and conjunctiva, including epithelial herpes simplex keratitis (dendritic keratitis), vaccinia, and varicella; mycobacterial infection of the eye and fungal diseases of the ocular structures; in patients with a known or suspected hypersensitivity to the product or any of its components or to other corticosteroids.

Warnings

Prolonged use of corticosteroids may result in glaucoma with damage to the optic nerve, defects in visual acuity and fields of vision, and posterior subcapsular cataract formation. Prolonged use of corticosteroids may suppress the host response and thus increase the hazard of secondary ocular infections. Various ocular diseases and long-term use of topical corticosteroids have been known to cause corneal and scleral thinning. Use of topical corticosteroids in the presence of thin corneal or scleral tissue may lead to perforation. Acute purulent infections of the eye may be masked or enhanced by the presence of corticosteroid medication. If this product is used for 10 days or longer, IOP should be routinely monitored even though it may be difficult in children and uncooperative patients. Steroids should be used with caution in the presence of glaucoma. IOP should be checked frequently. The use of steroids after cataract surgery may delay healing and increase the incidence of bleb formation. Use of ocular steroids may prolong the course and may exacerbate the severity of many viral infections of the eye (including herpes simplex). Employment of corticosteroid medication in the treatment of patients with a history of herpes simplex requires great caution; frequent slit-lamp microscopy is recommended.

Adverse Reactions

As fungal infections of the cornea are particularly prone to develop coincidentally with long-term corticosteroid applications, fungal invasion should be suspected in any persistent corneal ulceration where a corticosteroid has been used or is in use. Fungal cultures should be taken when appropriate. Reactions occurring most often from the presence of the anti-infective ingredient are allergic sensitizations. Reactions due to the steroid component in decreasing order of frequency are: elevation of IOP with possible development of glaucoma and infrequent optic nerve damage; posterior subcapsular cataract formation; delayed wound healing. Burning, stinging, and other symptoms of irritation have been reported with Pred-G. Superficial punctate keratitis has been reported occasionally, with onset occurring typically after several days of use.

Secondary infection: Has occurred after use of combinations containing steroids and antimicrobials. Fungal and viral infections of the cornea are particularly prone to develop coincidentally with long-term applications of steroid. The possibility of fungal invasion should be considered in any persistent corneal ulceration where steroid treatment has been used. Secondary bacterial ocular infection following suppression of host responses also occurs.

Pregnancy Category   C.

Glycerin

Brand Name   Refresh Endura.
Class of Drug   Lubricant eye drops.
Indications   Temporary relief of burning, irritation, and discomfort due to dryness of the eye or exposure to wind or sun. May be used as a protectant against further irritation.
Dosage Form   Active ingredients: glycerin 1% and polysorbate 80 1%. Available in preservative-free, disposable, single-use containers.
Dose   1–2 drops to affected eye(s) as needed and discard container.
Contraindications   In patients with a known hypersensitivity to the product or any of its components.
Warnings   For external use only. Stop use and ask a doctor if you experience eye pain, changes in vision, continued redness or irritation of the eye, or if the condition worsens or persists for more than 72 h.
Pregnancy Category C.

Brand Name   Tears Naturale Forte.
Class of Drug   Lubricant eye drops.
Indications   Temporary relief of burning and irritation due to dryness of the eye and for use as a protectant against further irritation. Temporary relief of discomfort due to minor irritations of the eye or to exposure to wind or sun.
Dosage Form   Active ingredients: dextran 70 0.1%, glycerin 0.2%, and hydroxypropyl methylcellulose 0.3%. Available in preservative-free reclosable vials.
Dose   1 or 2 drops to affected eye(s) as needed.
Contraindications   Known hypersensitivity to the product of any of its components.
Warnings   See »Refresh Endura.«
Pregnancy Category C.

Brand Name   Visine For Contacts Lubricating and Rewetting Drops.

Class of Drug	Lubricant eye drops.
Indications	May be used with daily- and extended-wear soft (hydrophilic) contact lenses for the following: moistening of daily-wear soft lenses while on the eyes during the day; moistening of extended-wear soft lenses upon awakening and as needed during the day; moistening of extended-wear soft lenses prior to retiring at night.
Dosage Form	Sterile, isotonic solution with a borate buffer system, hypromellose, and glycerin, with potassium sorbate and edetate disodium as the preservatives.
Dose	May be used as needed throughout the day.
Contraindications	In patients with known hypersensitivity to the product or any of its components.
Warnings	If minor irritation, discomfort, or blurring occurs while wearing lenses, place 1 or 2 drops on the eye and blink two or three times. If discomfort continues, immediately remove lenses and immediately see your eye care professional.
Adverse Reactions	May occur while wearing contact lenses: stinging, burning ,or itching (irritation); excessive watering (tearing); unusual secretions; redness; reduced sharpness of vision (visual acuity); blurred vision; sensitivity to light (photophobia); dry eyes.
Pregnancy Category	C.
Brand Name	Visine Tears; Visine Tears Preservative Free.
Class of Drug	Lubricant eye drops.
Indications	Temporary relief of burning and irritation due to dryness of the eye or protection against further irritation.
Dosage Form	Active ingredients: glycerin 0.2%, hypromellose 0.2%, and polyethylene glycol 400 1%. Available in preservative-free, single-use container.
Dose	1 or 2 drops to affected eye(s) as needed.
Contraindications	In patients with a known hypersensitivity to the product or any of its components.
Pregnancy Category	C.

Glycerin

Brand Name	Glycerin.
Class of Drug	Topical osmotic agent.
Indications	To clear an edematous cornea in order to facilitate ophthalmoscopic and gonioscopic examination, especially in acute glaucoma, bullous keratitis, Fuchs' endothelial dystrophy, etc. In gonioscopy of an edematous cornea, additional glycerin may be used as the lubricant. A local anesthetic should be instilled shortly before use of glycerin.

Dosage Form	Topical ophthalmic solution.
Dose	1 or 2 drops prior to examination. In gonioscopy of an edematous cornea, additional glycerin may be used as the lubricant.
Contraindications	In patients with hypersensitivity to the product or any of its components.
Adverse Reactions	Because glycerin is an irritant and may cause pain, a local anesthetic should be instilled shortly before its use.
Pregnancy Category	C.
Brand Name	Osmoglyn; Glyrol.
Class of Drug	Glaucoma. Oral osmotic agent.
Indications	Short-term reduction of IOP. May be used prior to and after intraocular surgery. May be used to interrupt an acute attack of glaucoma.
Dosage Form	Oral solution. Glycerin 50% (volume/volume).
Dose	2–3 ml/kg of body weight (approximately 4–6 oz. per individual) given as a single dose. Serving over cracked ice with a soda straw improves palatability.
Contraindications	In patients with well-established anuria, severe dehydration, frank or impending acute pulmonary edema, severe cardiac decompensation, and those with hypersensitivity to the product or any of its components.
Warnings	For oral use only. <u>Not for injection</u>. Caution should be exercised in hypervolemia, confused mental status, and congestive heart disease, and in the dehydrated patient, e.g., certain diabetics. Should be administered with caution to patients with cardiac, renal, or hepatic diseases. Altered hydration may lead to pulmonary edema and/or congestive heart failure.
Adverse Reactions	Nausea, vomiting, headaches, confusion, and disorientation may occur. Severe dehydration, cardiac arrhythmia, or hyperosmolar nonketotic coma, which can result in death, have been report.
Pregnancy Category	C.
Drug Interactions	Should be given to a pregnant woman only if clearly needed.

Gramicidin

Brand Name	Neosporin; Neomycin; Polymyxin B Sulfates; Gramicidin.
Class of Drug	Antibiotic, bactericidal. *Neomycin*: inhibits protein synthesis by binding with ribosomal RNA. *Polymyxin B*: increases permeability of bacterial cell membrane. *Gramicidin*: increases permeability of bacterial cell membrane to inorganic cations

by forming a network of channels through the normal lipid bilayer of the membrane.

Indications Topical treatment of superficial infections of the external eye and its adnexa caused by susceptible bacteria. Such infections encompass conjunctivitis, keratitis and keratoconjunctivitis, blepharitis and blepharoconjunctivitis. Neomycin sulfate, polymyxin B sulfate, and gramicidin together are considered active against the following microorganisms:*S. aureus;* streptococci, including *S. pneumoniae; E. coli; H. influenzae; Klebsiella* and *Enterobacter* spp.; *Neisseria* spp.; and *P. aeruginosa.* Does not provide adequate coverage against *S. marcescens.*

Dosage Form Ophthalmic solution: each milliliter contains neomycin sulfate (equivalent to 1.75 mg neomycin base), polymyxin B sulfate (equivalent to 10,000 polymyxin B units), and gramicidin 0.025 mg.

Dose 1 or 2 drops to affected eye(s) every 4 h for 7–10 days. In severe infections, dosage may be increased to as much as 2 drops every hour.

Contraindications In patients who have shown hypersensitivity to the product or any of its components.

Warnings Should never be directly introduced into anterior chamber of the eye or injected subconjunctivally. Topical antibiotics, particularly neomycin sulfate, may cause cutaneous sensitization. Manifestations of sensitization to topical antibiotics are usually itching, reddening, and edema of the conjunctiva and eyelid. A sensitization reaction may manifest simply as a failure to heal. During long-term use of topical antibiotic products, periodic examination for such signs is advisable, and the patient should be told to discontinue the product if they are observed. Symptoms usually subside quickly on withdrawing the medication. Applications of products containing these ingredients should be avoided for the patient thereafter.

Adverse Reactions As with other antibiotic preparations, prolonged use may result in overgrowth of nonsusceptible organisms, including fungi. If superinfection occurs, appropriate measures should be initiated. Bacterial resistance may also develop. If purulent discharge, inflammation, or pain becomes aggravated, the patient should discontinue use of the medication and consult a physician. Reactions occurring most often are allergic reactions, including itching, swelling, and conjunctival erythema. More serious hypersensitivity reactions, including anaphylaxis, have been reported rarely. Allergic cross-reactions may occur, which could prevent the use of any or all of the following antibiotics for the treatment of future infections: kanamycin, paromomycin, streptomycin, and possibly gentamicin.

Pregnancy Category C.

Homatropine Hydrobromide

Brand Name	Isopto Homatropine.
Class of Drug	Anticholinergic, mydriatic, cycloplegic.
Indications	Moderately long-acting mydriatic and cycloplegic for refraction and in the treatment of inflammatory conditions of the uveal tract. For pre- and postoperative states when mydriasis is required. Use as an optical aid in some cases of axial lens opacities.
Dosage Form	Topical ophthalmic solution 2% or 5%.
Dose	*Refraction*: 1–2 drops topically in the eye(s); may be repeated in 5–10 min if necessary. *Uveitis*: 1–2 drops topically up to every 3–4 h; individuals with heavily pigmented irides may require larger doses. Only the 2% strength should be used in pediatric patients.
Contraindications	In the presence of an anatomic NAG or patients with primary glaucoma or a tendency toward glaucoma, and in patients hypersensitive to the product or any of its components, including the belladonna alkaloid group. To avoid inducing ACG, an estimation of the depth of the angle of the anterior chamber should be made.
Warnings	Risk–benefit should be considered when the following medical problems exist: keratoconus (homatropine may produce fixed dilated pupil), Down syndrome, children with brain damage, the elderly (increased susceptibility). In infants and small children, use with extreme caution. Excessive use in children or certain individuals with a history of susceptibility to belladonna alkaloids may produce systemic symptoms of homatropine poisoning.
Adverse Reactions	Prolonged use may produce local irritation characterized by follicular conjunctivitis, vascular congestion, edema, exudate, and eczematoid dermatitis. Systemic homatropine toxicity is manifested by flushing and dryness of the skin (a rash may be present in children), dryness of the mouth, anhidrosis, blurred vision, photophobia, loss of neuromuscular coordination (ataxic gait), rapid and irregular pulse, fever, abdominal and bladder distention, dysarthric quality of speech, and mental aberration (hallucinosis) with recovery frequently followed by retrograde amnesia. Excessive topical use can potentially lead to a confusional state characterized by delirium, agitation, and, rarely, coma. The specific antidote for this systemic anticholinergic syndrome is injectable physostigmine salicylate.
Pregnancy Category	C.

Hydrocortisone

Brand Name	Cortisporin; AK Spore HC (bacitracin zinc, hydrocortisone, neomycin, polymyxin B).
Class of Drug	See »Bacitracin, Cortisporin.«
Indications	See »Bacitracin, Cortisporin.«
Dosage Form	See »Bacitracin, Cortisporin.«
Dose	See »Bacitracin, Cortisporin.«
Contraindications	See »Bacitracin, Cortisporin.«
Warnings	See »Bacitracin, Cortisporin.«
Adverse Reactions	See »Bacitracin, Cortisporin.«
Pregnancy Category	See »Bacitracin, Cortisporin.«
Drug Interactions	See »Bacitracin, Cortisporin.«

Hydroxypropyl Cellulose

Brand Name	Lacrisert.
Class of Drug	Dry eye relief.
Indications	In patients with moderate to severe dry eye syndromes, including keratoconjunctivitis sicca. Also for patients with exposure keratitis, decreased corneal sensitivity, recurrent corneal erosions.
Dosage Form	Hydroxypropyl cellulose ophthalmic insert: sterile, translucent, rod-shaped, water soluble, for administration into the inferior cul-de-sac of the eye. Each insert is 5 mg of hydroxypropyl cellulose. Approximately 1.27 mm in diameter by 3.5 mm long.
Dose	One insert in each eye once per day is usually sufficient to relieve the symptoms associated with moderate to severe dry eye syndromes. Individual patients may require more flexibility in the use of Lacrisert; some patients may require two times per day use for optimal results.
Contraindications	In patients who are hypersensitive to the product or any of its components.
Warnings	Instructions for inserting and removing should be carefully followed. Because this product may produce transient blurring of vision, patients should be instructed to exercise caution when operating hazardous machinery or driving a motor vehicle.
Adverse Reactions	Transient blurring of vision, ocular discomfort or irritation, matting or stickiness of eyelashes, photophobia, hypersensitivity, edema of the eyelids, hyperemia.

Drug Interactions	Application to the eyes of unanesthetized rabbits immediately prior to or 2 h before instilling pilocarpine, proparacaine HCl (0.5%), or phenylephrine (5%) did not markedly alter the magnitude and/or duration of the miotic, local corneal anesthetic, or mydriatic activity, respectively, of these agents. Under various treatment schedules, the anti-inflammatory effect of ocularly instilled dexamethasone (0.1%) in unanesthetized rabbits with primary uveitis was not affected by the presence of hydroxypropyl cellulose inserts.

Hydroxypropyl Methylcellulose

Brand Name	Bion Tears.
Class of Drug	See »Dextran 70, Bion Tears.«
Indications	See »Dextran 70, Bion Tears.«
Dosage Form	See »Dextran 70, Bion Tears.«
Dose	See »Dextran 70, Bion Tears.«
Contraindications	In patients with a known hypersensitivity to the product or any of its components.
Warnings	See »Dextran 70, Bion Tears.«
Pregnancy Category	C.

Brand Name	GenTeal.
Class of Drug	Lubricant eye drops.
Indications	Dry eyes.
Dosage Form	Topical ophthalmic solution. Hydroxypropyl methylcellulose 0.3%.
Dose	1 or 2 drops to affected eye(s) as needed.
Contraindications	In patients with a known hypersensitivity to the product or any of its components.

Brand Name	GenTeal Gel.
Class of Drug	Lubricant gel.
Indications	Dry eyes.
Dosage Form	Topical ophthalmic ointment. Hydroxypropyl methylcellulose 0.3% gel. Contains a disappearing preservative that turns into pure water and oxygen upon contact with your eye.
Dose	1 or 2 drops to affected eye(s) as needed.
Contraindications	In patients with a known hypersensitivity to the product or any of its components.

Brand Name	GenTeal Mild.
Class of Drug	Lubricant eye drops.
Indications	Dry eyes.

Dosage Form	Topical ophthalmic solution. Hydroxypropyl methylcellulose 0.2%. Contain a disappearing preservative that turns into pure water and oxygen upon contact with your eye.
Dose	1 or 2 drops to affected eye(s) as needed.
Contraindications	In patients with a known hypersensitivity to the product or any of its components.

Brand Name	GenTeal PF.
Class of Drug	Lubricant eye drops.
Indications	Dry eyes.
Dosage Form	Topical ophthalmic solution. Hydroxypropyl methylcellulose 0.2%. Preservative free.
Dose	1 or 2 drops to affected eye(s) as needed.
Contraindications	In patients with a known hypersensitivity to the product or any of its components.

Hydroxypropyl Methylcellulose

Brand Name	Goniosol.
Class of Drug	Diagnostic aid.
Indications	Lubrication during ophthalmic examination.
Dosage Form	Ophthalmic solution 2.5%.
Dose	Provide lubrication between diagnostic instrument and surface of eye.
Contraindications	In patients with a known hypersensitivity to the product or any of its components.

Brand Name	Ocucoat.
Class of Drug	Isotonic nonpyrogenic viscoelastic.
Indications	For use as an ophthalmic surgical aid in anterior segment surgical procedures, including cataract extraction and intraocular lens (IOL) implantation. Maintains the anterior chamber during cataract surgery and thereby allows for more efficient manipulation with less trauma to the corneal endothelium and other ocular tissues.
Dosage Form	Injectable. Hydroxypropyl methylcellulose 2%.
Dose	In anterior segment surgery, may be injected into the chamber prior to or following delivery of the crystalline lens. Injection prior to lens delivery will provide additional protection to the corneal endothelium and other ocular tissues. May also be used to coat an IOL as well as tips of surgical instruments prior to implantation surgery. Additional dose may be injected during anterior segment surgery to fully maintain the chamber or to replace fluid lost during the surgical procedure. Should be removed from the anterior chamber at the

end of surgery: Rather than aspirate from the eye with the Ocucoat syringe, it is recommended it be aspirated using an automated irrigation and aspiration device or irrigated using an irrigation syringe or a BSS squeeze bottle.

Contraindications   In patients with a known hypersensitivity to the product or any of its components.

Adverse Reactions   *Precautions*: Limited to those normally associated with the ophthalmic surgical procedure being performed. There may be transient increased IOP following surgery because of preexisting glaucoma or due to the surgery itself. For these reasons, the following precautions should be considered: Ocucoat should be removed from the anterior chamber at the end of surgery. If postoperative IOP increases above expected values, appropriate therapy should be administered. *Adverse reactions*: Clinical testing showed it to be extremely well tolerated after injection into the human eye. A transient rise in IOP postoperatively has been reported in some cases. Rarely, postoperative inflammatory reactions (iritis, hypopyon), as well as incidents of corneal edema and corneal decompensation, have been reported with viscoelastic agents; their relationship to Ocucoat has not been established.

Brand Name	Tears Naturale Forte.
Class of Drug	Lubricant eye drops.
Indications	See »Dextran 70, Tears Naturale Forte.«
Dosage Form	See »Dextran 70, Tears Naturale Forte.«
Dose	See »Dextran 70, Tears Naturale Forte.«
Contraindications	In patients with a known hypersensitivity to the product or any of its components.
Warnings	See »Dextran 70, Tears Naturale Forte.«
Pregnancy Category	

Brand Name	Tear Naturale Free.
Class of Drug	Lubricant eye drops.
Indications	See »Dextran 70, Tear Naturale Free.«
Dosage Form	See »Dextran 70, Tear Naturale Free.«
Dose	See »Dextran 70, Tear Naturale Free.«
Contraindications	In patients with a known hypersensitivity to the product or any of its components.
Warnings	See »Dextran 70, Tear Naturale Free.«

Brand Name	Visine For Contacts Rewetting.
Class of Drug	Lubricant eye drops.
Indications	See »Glycerin, Visine For Contacts Lubricating and Rewetting Drops.«
Dosage Form	See »Glycerin, Visine For Contacts Lubricating and Rewetting Drops.«
Dose	See »Glycerin, Visine For Contacts Lubricating and Rewetting Drops.«

Contraindications	In patients with a known hypersensitivity to the product or any of its components.
Warnings	See »Glycerin, Visine For Contacts Lubricating and Rewetting Drops.«
Adverse Reactions	See »Glycerin, Visine For Contacts Lubricating and Rewetting Drops.«
Pregnancy Category	C.

Hypromellose

Brand Name	Visine Tears.
Class of Drug	Lubricant eye drops.
Indications	See »Glycerin, Visine Tears.«
Dosage Form	See »Glycerin, Visine Tears.«
Dose	See »Glycerin, Visine Tears.«
Contraindications	In patients with a known hypersensitivity to the product or any of its components.
Pregnancy Category	

Brand Name	Visine Tears Preservative-Free.
Class of Drug	Lubricant eye drops.
Indications	See »Glycerin, Visine Tears Preservative-Free.«
Dosage Form	See »Glycerin Visine Tears Preservative-Free.«
Dose	See »Glycerin Visine Tears Preservative-Free.«
Contraindications	In patients with a known hypersensitivity to the product or any of its components.

Imipenem/Cilastatin Sodium

Brand Name — Primaxin.

Class of Drug — Antibiotic.

Indications — LRIs—*S. aureus* (penicillinase-producing strains), *Acinetobacter* spp., *Enterobacter* spp., *E. coli*, *H. influenzae*, *Haemophilus parainfluenzae**, *Klebsiella* spp., *S. marcescens*. UTIs (complicated and uncomplicated)—*Enterococcus faecalis*, *S. aureus* (penicillinase-producing strains)*, *Enterobacter* spp., *E. coli*, *Klebsiella* spp., *M. morganii**, *P. vulgaris**, *Providencia rettgeri**, *P. aeruginosa*. Intra-abdominal infections—*E. faecalis*; *S. aureus* (penicillinase-producing strains)*; *S. epidermidis*; *Citrobacter* spp.; *Enterobacter* spp.; *E. coli*; *Klebsiella* spp.; *M. morganii**; *Proteus* spp.; *P. aeruginosa*; *Bifidobacterium* spp.; *Clostridium* spp.; *Eubacterium* spp.; *Peptococcus* spp.; *Peptostreptococcus* spp.; *Propionibacterium* spp.*; *Bacteroides* spp., including *B. fragilis*; *Fusobacterium* spp. Gynecologic infections—*E. faecalis*; *S. aureus* (penicillinase-producing strains)*; *S. epidermidis*; *Streptococcus agalactiae* (group B streptococci); *Enterobacter* spp.*; *E. coli*; *Gardnerella vaginalis*; *Klebsiella* spp.*; *Proteus* spp.; *Bifidobacterium* spp.*; *Peptococcus* spp.*; *Peptostreptococcus* spp.; *Propionibacterium* spp.*; *Bacteroides* spp., including *B. fragilis**; bacterial septicemia; *E. faecalis*; *S. aureus* (penicillinase-producing strains); *Enterobacter* spp.; *E. coli*; *Klebsiella* spp.; *P. aeruginosa*; *Serratia* spp.*;Bone and joint infections—*E. faecalis*, *S. aureus* (penicillinase-producing strains), *S. epidermidis*, *Enterobacter* spp., *P. aeruginosa*. Skin and skin structure infections—*E. faecalis*; *S. aureus* (penicillinase-producing strains); *S. epidermidis*; *Acinetobacter* spp.; *Citrobacter* spp.; *Enterobacter* spp.; *E. coli*; *Klebsiella* spp.; *M. morganii*; *P. vulgaris*; *P. rettgeri**; *P. aeruginosa*; *Serratia* spp.; *Peptococcus* spp.; *Peptostreptococcus* spp.; *Bacteroides* spp., including *B. fragilis*; *Fusobacterium* spp.*. Endocarditis—*S. aureus* (penicillinase-producing strains). Polymicrobic infections—Primaxin i.v. is indicated for polymicrobic infections, including those in which *S. pneumoniae* (pneumonia, septicemia), *S. pyogenes* (skin and skin structure), or non-penicillinase-producing *S. aureus* is one of the causative organisms. However, monobacterial infections due to these organisms are usually treated with narrower spectrum antibiotics, such as penicillin G.

Dosage Form Dose — *Adult minimum:maxixum*: 1,000.0 mg:4000.0 mg. *Pediatric minimum:maximum*: 60.0 mg/kg:100.0 mg/kg. Total daily dosage should be based on the type or severity of infection and given in equally divided doses based on consideration of degree of susceptibility of the pathogen(s), renal function, and body weight. *Adult patients*: with impaired renal function, as judged by CrCl ≤70 ml/min per 1.73 m^2 require adjustment of dosage. *Pediatric patients 3 months of* *age or older*: recommended dose for non-CNS infections is 15–25 mg/kg per dose every 6 h; based on studies in adults, maximum daily dose for treatment of infections with fully susceptible organisms is 2.0 g per day and of infections with moderately susceptible organisms (primarily some strains of *P. aeruginosa*) is 4.0 g/day; higher doses (up to 90 mg/kg per day in older children) have been used in patients with cystic fibrosis. *Pediatric patients 3 months of age or less (weighing ≥1,500 g)*: recommended dosage schedule for non-CNS infections: younger than 1 week of age—25 mg/kg every 12 h; 1–4 weeks of age—25 mg/kg every 8 h; 4 weeks to 3 months of age—25 mg/kg every 6 h.

Contraindications

In patients who have shown hypersensitivity to the product or any of its components or with CNS disorder or renal disease.

Warnings

Not recommended in pediatric patients with CNS infections because of the risk of seizures. Not recommended in pediatric patients <30 kg with impaired renal function as no data are available.*CNS*: including confusional states, myoclonic activity, and seizures have been reported, especially when recommended dosages were exceeded. These experiences have occurred most commonly in patients with CNS disorders (e.g., brain lesions or history of seizures) and/or compromised renal function. However, there have been reports of CNS adverse experiences in patients who had no recognized or documented underlying CNS disorder or compromised renal function. When recommended doses were exceeded, adult patients with CrCl of ≤20 ml/min per 1.73 m^2, whether or not undergoing hemodialysis, had a higher risk of seizure activity than those without impairment of renal function. Therefore, close adherence to dosing guidelines for these patients is recommended. Patients with CrCl of ≤5 ml/min per 1.73 m^2 should not receive Primaxin i.v. unless hemodialysis is instituted within 48 h. For patients on hemodialysis, Primaxin i.v. is recommended only when the benefit outweighs the potential risk of seizures. Close adherence to the recommended dosage and dosage schedules is urged, especially in patients with known risk factors that predispose to convulsive activity. Anticonvulsant therapy should be continued in patients with known seizure disorders. If focal tremors, myoclonus, or seizures occur, patients should be evaluated neurologically, placed on anticonvulsant therapy if not already instituted, and the dosage of Primaxin i.v. re-examined to determine whether it should be decreased or discontinued.

Serious and occasionally fatal hypersensitivity (anaphylactic) reactions have been reported in patients receiving therapy with beta-lactams. These reactions are more apt to occur in persons with a history of sensitivity to multiple allergens.

There have been reports of patients with a history of penicillin hypersensitivity who experienced severe hypersensitivity reactions when treated with another beta-lactam. Before initiating therapy with Primaxin i.v., careful inquiry should be made concerning previous hypersensitivity reactions to penicillins, cephalosporins, other beta-lactams, and other allergens. If an allergic reaction occurs, Primaxin should be discontinued. Serious anaphylactic reactions require immediate emergency treatment with epinephrine. Oxygen, intravenous steroids, and airway management, including intubation, may also be administered as indicated.

Adverse Reactions   *Most frequent*: allergic reactions, CNS toxicity, diarrhea, drug fever, gastrointestinal disorder, nausea, pruritus, skin rash, thrombophlebitis, urticaria, vomiting, wheezing. *Rare*: C. difficile colitis.

Pregnancy Category C.

Drug Interactions   It is not known whether this drug is excreted in human milk. Use in pediatric patients—neonates to 16 years of age—is supported by evidence from adequate and well-controlled studies in adults and by clinical studies and published literature in pediatric patients.

Indocyanine Green

Brand Name   IC-Green.
Class of Drug   Diagnostic and therapeutic aid.
Indications   Ophthalmic diagnostic angiography; intraoperative. Staining of anterior capsule in cataract surgery; staining of internal limiting membrane in macular surgery.
Dosage Form   Powder for injection 25 mg (10 ml of aqueous solvent provided). A sterile, water soluble, tricarbocyanine dye with a peak spectral absorption at 800–810 nm in blood plasma or blood. Contains up to 5% sodium iodide.
Dose   *Ophthalmic diagnostic angiography*: dissolve 25 mg of IC-Green with 5 ml of aqueous solvent provided through filter. Inject the 5 ml solution intravenously over approximately 10 s as a bolus. *Intraoperative*: add 1 ml solvent and 4 ml BSS to 25-mg vial of IC-Green powder; deliver 1 ml of the dissolved solution to the sterile field though filter to be used intraoperatively. Dissolved solution can be further diluted by mixing with BSS. Unstable in aqueous solution and must be used within 10 h after preparation. However, the dye is stable in plasma and whole blood so that samples obtained in discontinuous sampling techniques may be read hours later. Sterile techniques should be used in handling the dye

solution as well as in the performance of the dilution curves.

Contraindications Contains sodium iodide, and should be used with caution in patients who have a history of allergy to iodides.

Warnings Two anaphylactic deaths have been reported following administration during cardiac catheterization. One was in a patient with a history of sensitivity to penicillin and sulfa drugs. The aqueous solvent provided with this product, pH 5.5–6.5, which is specially prepared sterile water for injection, should be used to dissolve indocyanine green because there have been reports of incompatibility with some commercially available water for injection.

Adverse Reactions Powder may cling to the vial or lump together because it is freeze-dried in the vials. This is not due to the presence of water. Anaphylactic or urticarial reactions have been reported in patients with or without history of allergy to iodides; if such reactions occur, treatment with the appropriate agents, e.g., epinephrine, antihistamines, and corticosteroids, should be administered.

Pregnancy Category C.

Drug Interactions Plasma fractional disappearance rate at the recommended 0.5 mg/kg dose has been reported to be significantly greater in women than in men; however, there was no significant difference in the calculated value for clearance. Radioactive iodine uptake studies should not be performed for at least a week following the use of indocyanine green. Heparin preparations containing sodium bisulfite reduce the absorption peak of indocyanine green in blood. Do not use heparin as an anticoagulant for the collection of samples for analysis.

Infliximab

Brand Name Remicade.

Class of Drug Neutralizes biological activity of TNF-alpha by binding with high affinity to soluble and transmembrane forms of TNF-alpha and inhibits binding of TNF-alpha with its receptors.

Indications Rheumatoid arthritis that has an inadequate response to methotrexate; Crohn's disease that has an inadequate response to conventional therapy. *Off-label*: refractory posterior uveitis, Behçet disease panuveitis, recurrent anterior uveitis.

Dosage Form Powder for i.v. injection 100 mg/20 ml.

Dose 3–10 mg/kg i.v. every 4–8 weeks.

Contraindications In patients with a known hypersensitivity to the product or any of its components.

Warnings	Serious and potentially fatal infections and sepsis have occurred in the setting of TNF-alpha blockade, including histoplasmosis, listeriosis, and pneumocystosis. Has been associated with hypersensitivity reactions that vary in their time of onset; most hypersensitivity reactions, which include urticaria, dyspnea, and/or hypotension, have occurred during or within 2 h of infusion.
Adverse Reactions	Opportunistic infections after prolonged use; TB reactivations; injection-related hypersensitivity, including urticaria, dyspnea, and hypotension; new onset or exacerbation of preexisting CNS demyelinating disorders; autoantibodies/Lupus-like syndrome. Reports of new occurrence of non-Hodgkin's B-cell lymphoma, breast cancer, melanoma, squamous, rectal adenocarcinoma, and basal cell carcinoma have been described; insufficient data to determine whether infliximab contributed to the development of these malignancies. Rule out prior TB infection with PPD and CXR. Monitor CBC with differential, ALT, and AST every 2 weeks for first month, then every 4–6 weeks.
Pregnancy Category	B.
Drug Interactions	Safety and effectiveness in patients with JRA and pediatric patients with Crohn's disease have not been established. Concurrent administration of etanercept and anakinra (an IL-1 antagonist) has been associated with an increased risk of serious infections and increased risk of neutropenia and no additional benefit compared with these products alone. Other TNF-alpha-blocking agents used in combination with anakinra may also result in similar toxicities.

Interferon alpha-2a (IFN-alpha 2a)

Brand Name	Roferon A.
Class of Drug	Antiviral. Decreases activity of natural killer cells.
Indications	Various hematologic malignancies, chronic viral infections, Kaposi sarcoma. *Off-label*: uveitis refractory, in the setting of Behçet disease.
Dosage Form	Solution injectable for subcutaneous or i.m. injection: 3 million units/0.5 ml, 6 million units/0.5 ml, 9 million units/0.5 ml, 36 million units/0.5 ml.
Dose	3–9 million units three times per week.
Contraindications	In patients with a known hypersensitivity to the product or any of its components. Injectable solutions contain benzyl alcohol and are contraindicated in any individual with a known allergy to that preservative.
Warnings	Depression and suicidal behavior have been reported. *CNS*: Reported in a number of patients, including decreased men-

tal status, dizziness, impaired memory, agitation, manic behavior, and psychotic reactions. More severe obtundation and coma have been rarely observed. Most were mild and reversible within a few days to 3 weeks upon dose reduction or discontinuation of therapy. Careful periodic neuropsychiatric monitoring of all patients is recommended. *Cardiac*: Should be administered with caution to patients with cardiac disease or with any history of cardiac illness. Acute, self-limited toxicities (i.e., fever, chills) frequently associated with administration may exacerbate preexisting cardiac conditions. Rarely, myocardial infarction has occurred cases and cardiomyopathy observed. *Hepatic*: Patients with a history of autoimmune hepatitis or autoimmune disease and patients who are immunosuppressed transplant recipients should not be treated with INF-alpha-2a. In chronic hepatitis C, initiation of therapy has been reported to cause transient liver abnormalities, which in patients with poorly compensated liver disease can result in increased ascites, hepatic failure, or death. Leukopenia and elevation of hepatic enzymes occurred frequently but were rarely dose limiting. Thrombocytopenia occurred less frequently. Proteinuria and increased cells in urinary sediment were also seen infrequently. *Other*: Infrequently, severe renal toxicities, sometimes requiring renal dialysis, have been reported with IFN-alpha therapy alone or in combination with IL-2. Infrequently, severe or fatal gastrointestinal hemorrhage has been reported. Caution should be exercised when administering to patients with myelosuppression or when used in combination with other agents known to cause myelosuppression. Synergistic toxicity has been observed when administered in combination with zidovudine (AZT). Hyperglycemia has been observed rarely; patients with diabetes mellitus may require adjustment of their antidiabetic regimen. Should not be used for the treatment of visceral AIDS-related Kaposi's sarcoma associated with rapidly progressive or life-threatening disease.

Adverse Reactions   Increased risk of TB reactivation, leukopenia, thrombocytopenia, severe depression, flu-like symptoms, erythema at injection site, alopecia, gastrointestinal upset. Monitor CBC with differential, ALT, and AST every 2 weeks for first month then every 4–6 weeks; periodic ophthalmologic examination to rule out interferon retinopathy as well as psychiatric examination.

Pregnancy Category   C.

Drug Interactions   In children with Ph-positive adult-type CML is supported by evidence from adequate and well-controlled studies of interferon alfa-2a in adults with additional data from the literature on the use of alpha interferon in children with chronic myelogenous leukemia (CML).

Itraconazole

Brand Name   Sporanox.
Class of Drug   Antifungal.
Indications   Empiric therapy of febrile neutropenic patients with sus-
                       pected fungal infections. Injection is also indicated for the
                       treatment of the following fungal infections in immunocom-
                       promised and nonimmunocompromised patients: blastomy-
                       cosis, pulmonary and extrapulmonary; histoplasmosis, inclu-
                       ding chronic cavitary pulmonary disease and disseminated,
                       nonmeningeal histoplasmosis; aspergillosis, pulmonary and
                       extrapulmonary, in patients who are intolerant of or who are
                       refractory to amphotericin B therapy.
Dosage Form   Injection, capsule, solution.
Dose   *Empiric therapy in febrile, neutropenic patients with suspected*
                       fungal infections (ETFN): IV 200 mg two times per day for four
                       doses, followed by 200 mg once per day for up to 14 days.
                       Each i.v. dose should be infused over 1 h. Treatment should
                       be continued with oral solution 200 mg (20 ml) two times per
                       day until resolution of clinically significant neutropenia. *Blas-*
                       tomycosis, histoplasmosis, and aspergillosis: IV or p.o. 200 mg
                       two times per day for four doses, followed by 200 mg q.d.
                       Each i.v. dose should be infused over 1 h. Total itraconazole
                       therapy (injection followed by oral) should be continued for
                       a minimum of 3 months and until clinical parameters and
                       laboratory tests indicate that the active fungal infection has
                       subsided. An inadequate period of treatment may lead to re-
                       currence of active infection. Injection should not be used in
                       patients with CrCl <30 ml/min.
Contraindications In patients who have shown hypersensitivity to the product
                       or any of its components . Caution should be used when
                       prescribing to patients with hypersensitivity to other azoles.
                       Life-threatening cardiac dysrhythmias and/or sudden death
                       have occurred in patients using cisapride, pimozide, leva-
                       cetylmethadol (levomethadyl), or quinidine concomitantly
                       with Sporanox and/or other CYP3A4 inhibitors. Concomitant
                       administration of these drugs with Sporanox is contraindica-
                       ted.
Warnings   *Hepatic effects*: rare cases of serious hepatotoxicity, including
                       liver failure and death, have been reported. *Cardiac dysrhyth-*
                       mias: life-threatening cardiac dysrhythmias and/or sudden
                       death have occurred in patients using cisapride, pimozide,
                       levacetylmethadol (levomethadyl), or quinidine concomi-
                       tantly with Sporanox and/or other CYP3A4 inhibitors. *Car-*
                       diac disease: injection should not be used in patients with
                       evidence of ventricular dysfunction unless the benefit clearly
                       outweighs the risk. Injection contains the excipient hydroxy-

propyl-(beta)-cyclodextrin, which produced pancreatic adenocarcinomas in a rat carcinogenicity study. These findings were not observed in a similar mouse carcinogenicity study. The clinical relevance of these findings is unknown.

Adverse Reactions

Rare: severe hepatotoxicity. *Postmarketing*: events of gastrointestinal origin, such as dyspepsia, nausea, vomiting, diarrhea, abdominal pain, and constipation. Also, congenital abnormalities, including skeletal, genitourinary tract, cardiovascular, and ophthalmic malformations, as well as chromosomal and multiple malformations, have been reported but a causal relationship has not been established *Other*: includes peripheral edema, congestive heart failure, and pulmonary edema, headache, dizziness, peripheral neuropathy, menstrual disorders, reversible increases in hepatic enzymes, hepatitis, liver failure, hypokalemia, hypertriglyceridemia, alopecia, allergic reactions (such as pruritus, rash, urticaria, angioedema, anaphylaxis), Stevens–Johnson syndrome, anaphylactic, anaphylactoid and allergic reactions, photosensitivity and neutropenia.

Pregnancy Category

C.

Drug Interactions

Itraconazole and its major metabolite, hydroxyitraconazole, are inhibitors of CYP3A4 and may decrease the elimination of drugs metabolized by CYP3A4, resulting in increased plasma concentrations of these drugs. Inducers or inhibitors of CYP3A4 may decrease or increase the plasma concentrations of itraconazole. The class IA antiarrhythmic quinidine and class III antiarrhythmic dofetilide are known to prolong the QT interval. Coadministration of quinidine or dofetilide with itraconazole may increase plasma concentrations of both drugs, which could result in serious cardiovascular events. Therefore, concomitant administration of itraconazole and quinidine or dofetilide is contraindicated. Concomitant administration of digoxin and itraconazole has led to increased plasma concentrations of digoxin. Itraconazole enhances the anticoagulant effect of coumarin-like drugs, such as warfarin. The following drugs can have plasma concentrations increased by itraconazole: Disopyramide, carbamazepine, rifabutin, busulfan, docetaxel, vinca alkaloids, pimozide, alprazolam, diazepam, midazolam, triazolam, dihydropyridine, verapamil, cisapride, atorvastatin, cerivastatin, lovastatin, simvastatin, cyclosporine, tacrolimus, sirolimus, oral hypoglycemics, indinavir, ritonavir, saquinavir, levacetylmethadol, levomethadyl, ergot alkaloids, halofantrine, alfentanil, buspirone, methylprednisolone, budesonide, dexamethasone, trimetrexate, warfarin, cilostazol, eletriptan.

Ketoconazole

Brand Name Nizoral.

Class of Drug Antifungal.

Indications *Systemic fungal infections*: candidiasis, chronic mucocutaneous candidiasis, oral thrush, candiduria, blastomycosis, coccidioidomycosis, histoplasmosis, chromomycosis, and paracoccidioidomycosis; fungal endophthalmitis. Tablets should not be used for fungal meningitis because it penetrates poorly into the cerebral spinal fluid. *Severe recalcitrant cutaneous dermatophyte infections*: tablets are also indicated for patients who have not responded to topical therapy or oral griseofulvin or who are unable to take griseofulvin.

Dosage Form Oral tablet.

Dose *Adults*: Starting dose is a single daily administration of 200 mg (1 tablet). In very serious infections or if clinical responsiveness is insufficient within the expected time, dose may be increased to 400 mg (1 tablets) once per day. *Children*: In small numbers of children older than 2 years of age, a single daily dose of 3.3–6.6 mg/kg has been used. Tablets have not been studied in children younger than 2 years of age.

Minimum treatment for candidiasis is 1 or 2 weeks. Patients with chronic mucocutaneous candidiasis usually require maintenance therapy. Minimum treatment for the other indicated systemic mycoses is 6 months. Minimum treatment for recalcitrant dermatophyte infections is 4 weeks in cases involving glabrous skin. Palmar and plantar infections may respond more slowly. Apparent cures may subsequently recur after discontinuation of therapy in some cases.

Contraindications Coadministration with terfenadine, cisapride, astemizole, or oral triazolam. Coadministration with terfenadine has led to elevated plasma concentrations of terfenadine, which may prolong QT intervals, sometimes resulting in life-threatening cardiac dysrhythmias. Cases of *torsades de pointes* and other serious ventricular dysrhythmias, in rare cases leading to fatality, have been reported among patients taking terfenadine concurrently with ketoconazole tablets. Concomitant administration with cisapride because it has resulted in markedly elevated cisapride plasma concentrations and prolonged QT interval and has rarely been associated with ventricular arrhythmias and *torsades de pointes*. In patients who have shown hypersensitivity to the product or any of its components.

Warnings Hepatotoxicity, primarily of the hepatocellular type, including rare fatalities. Several cases of hepatitis have been reported in children. LFTs (such as SGGT, alkaline phosphatase, SGPT, SGOT, and bilirubin) should be measured before starting treatment and at frequent intervals during treatment. Patients should be instructed to report any signs and symptoms that may suggest liver dysfunction so that appropriate biochemical testing can be done. Such signs and symptoms may include unusual fatigue, anorexia, nausea and/or vomiting, jaundice, dark urine, or pale stools. In rare cases, anaphylaxis has been reported after the first dose. Several cases of hypersensitivity reactions, including urticaria, have also been reported. High doses are known to suppress adrenal corticosteroid secretion. The recommended dose of 200–400 mg per day should be followed closely. Tablets require acidity for dissolution; if concomitant antacids, anticholinergics, and H_2 blockers are needed, they should be given at least 2 h after administration of Nizoral tablets. In cases of achlorhydria, patients should be instructed to dissolve each tablet in 4 ml aqueous solution of 0.2 N HCl. For ingesting the resulting mixture, they should use a drinking straw so as to avoid contact with the teeth. This administration should be followed with a cup of tap water.

Adverse Reactions
Most frequent: nausea and/or vomiting, abdominal pain, pruritus. *Less frequent*: headache, dizziness, somnolence, fever and chills, photophobia, diarrhea, gynecomastia, impotence, thrombocytopenia, leukopenia, hemolytic anemia, bulging fontanelles. *Rare*: alopecia; paresthesia; signs of increased intracranial pressure, including bulging fontanelles and papilledema; hypertriglyceridemia; neuropsychiatric disturbances, including suicidal tendencies and severe depression; in rare cases, anaphylaxis has been reported after the first dose; several cases of hypersensitivity reactions, including urticaria have also been reported; hepatic dysfunction is a rare occurrence. Testosterone levels are impaired with doses of 800 mg per day and abolished by 1,600 mg per day; once therapy has been discontinued, serum testosterone levels return to baseline values.

Pregnancy Category
C.

Drug Interactions
A potent inhibitor of the cytochrome P450 3A4 enzyme system. Coadministration with drugs primarily metabolized by the cytochrome P450 3A4 enzyme system may result in increased plasma concentrations of the drugs that could increase or prolong both therapeutic and adverse effects.

Ketorolac Tromethamine

Brand Name
Acular.

Class of Drug
NSAID.

Indications
For temporary relief of ocular itching due to seasonal allergic conjunctivitis; treatment of postoperative inflammation in patients who have undergone cataract extraction.

Dosage Form	Topical ophthalmic solution 0.5%.
Dose	1 drop four times per day for relief of ocular itching due to seasonal allergic conjunctivitis. For postoperative inflammation in patients who have undergone cataract extraction, 1 drop to the affected eye(s) four times per day beginning 24 h after cataract surgery and continuing through the first 2 weeks of the postoperative period.
Contraindications	In patients with previously demonstrated hypersensitivity to the product or any of its components.
Warnings	Potential for cross-sensitivity to acetylsalicylic acid, phenylacetic acid derivatives, and other nonsteroidal anti-inflammatory agents; therefore, caution should be used when treating individuals who have previously exhibited sensitivities to these drugs. With some NSAIDs, there exists the potential for increased bleeding time due to interference with thrombocyte aggregation. There have been reports that ocularly applied NSAIDs may cause increased bleeding of ocular tissues (including hyphemas) in conjunction with ocular surgery. All topical NSAIDs may slow or delay healing. Topical corticosteroids are also known to slow or delay healing. Concomitant use of topical NSAIDs and topical steroids may increase the potential for healing problems.
Adverse Reactions	Topical NSAIDs may result in keratitis. In some susceptible patients, continued use may result in epithelial breakdown, corneal thinning, corneal erosion, corneal ulceration, or corneal perforation; these events may be sight threatening. Patients with evidence of corneal epithelial breakdown should immediately discontinue use and should be closely monitored for corneal health. Postmarketing experience suggests that patients with complicated ocular surgeries, corneal denervation, corneal epithelial defects, diabetes mellitus, ocular surface diseases (e.g., dry eye syndrome), rheumatoid arthritis, or repeat ocular surgeries within a short period of time may be at increased risk for corneal adverse events, which may become sight threatening; should be used with caution in these patients. Use more than 24 h prior to surgery or beyond 14 days postsurgery may increase risk for occurrence and severity of corneal adverse events. It is recommended that Acular be used with caution in patients with known bleeding tendencies or who are receiving medications that may prolong bleeding time. Transient stinging and burning on instillation, allergic reactions, corneal edema, iritis, ocular inflammation, superficial keratitis, superficial ocular infections, corneal infiltrates, eye dryness, headaches, visual disturbance (blurry vision), and epithelial breakdown have been reported.
Pregnancy Category	C.
Brand Name	Acular LS.
Class of Drug	Topical NSAID.

Indications	Ophthalmic solution indicated for the reduction of ocular pain and burning/stinging following corneal refractive surgery.
Dosage Form	Topical ophthalmic solution 0.4%.
Dose	Recommended dose is 1 drop four times per day in the operated eye as needed for pain and burning/stinging for up to 4 days following corneal refractive surgery.
Contraindications	In patients with previously demonstrated hypersensitivity to the product or any of its components.
Warnings	See »Acular.«
Adverse Reactions	See »Acular.«
Pregnancy Category	See »Acular.«
Drug Interactions	See »Acular.«
Brand Name	Acular PF.
Class of Drug	Topical NSAID.
Indications	For the reduction of ocular pain and photophobia following incisional refractive surgery.
Dosage Form	Topical ophthalmic solution 0.5%. Preservative free.
Dose	1 drop four times per day in the operated eye as needed for pain and photophobia for up to 3 days after incisional refractive surgery.
Contraindications	In patients with previously demonstrated hypersensitivity to the product or any of its components.
Warnings	See »Acular.«
Adverse Reactions	See »Acular.«
Pregnancy Category	See »Acular.«
Drug Interactions	See »Acular.«

Ketotifen Fumarate

Brand Name	Zaditor.
Class of Drug	Relative selective, noncompetitive, histamine antagonist (H1-receptor) and mast cell stabilizer.
Indications	Temporary prevention of itching of the eye due to allergic conjunctivitis.
Dosage Form	Topical ophthalmic solution 0.025%.
Dose	1 drop to affected eye(s) two times per day every 8–12 h.
Contraindications	In persons with a known hypersensitivity to the product or any of its components.
Warnings	For topical ophthalmic use only. Not for injection or oral use.
Adverse Reactions	In controlled clinical studies, conjunctival infection, headaches, and rhinitis were reported at an incidence of 10–25%. Occurrences were generally mild; some were similar to the

underlying ocular disease being studied. The following ocular and nonocular adverse reactions were reported at an incidence of less than 5%:*Ocular*—allergic reactions, burning or stinging, conjunctivitis, discharge, dry eyes, eye pain, eyelid disorder, itching, keratitis, lacrimation disorder, mydriasis, photophobia, rash. *Nonocular*—flu syndrome, pharyngitis.

Pregnancy Category C.

Latanoprost

Brand Name	Xalatan.
Class of Drug	Glaucoma. Prostanoid-selective prostaglandin F (FP) receptor agonist.
Indications	Reduction of elevated IOP in patients with OAG or ocular hypertension.
Dosage Form	Topical ophthalmic solution 0.005% (50 μg/ml).
Dose	1 drop to affected eye(s) once per day in the evening; dosage should not exceed once per day since it has been shown that more frequent administration may decrease IOP-lowering effect. Reduction of IOP starts approximately 3–4 h after administration and the maximum effect is reached after 8–12 h.
Contraindications	In patients with known hypersensitivity to the product or any of its components or to benzalkonium chloride.
Warnings	Reported to cause changes to pigmented tissues. Most frequently reported changes have been increased pigmentation of the iris, periorbital tissue (eyelid) and eyelashes, and growth of eyelashes; pigmentation is expected to increase as long as Xalatan is administered. After discontinuation, pigmentation of the iris is likely to be permanent while pigmentation of the periorbital tissue and eyelash changes has been reported to be reversible in some patients. Patients who receive treatment should be informed of the possibility of increased pigmentation. The effects of increased pigmentation beyond 5 years are not known.
	May gradually increase pigmentation of the iris. The eye-color change is due to increased melanin content in the stromal melanocytes of the iris rather than to an increase in the number of melanocytes. This change may not be noticeable for several months to years Typically, the brown pigmentation around the pupil spreads concentrically toward the periphery of the iris, and the entire iris or parts of it become more brownish. Neither nevi nor freckles of the iris appear to be affected by treatment. While treatment can be continued in patients who develop noticeably increased iris pigmentation, these patients should be examined regularly. During clinical trials, the increase in brown iris pigment has not been shown to progress further upon discontinuation of treatment, but the resultant color change may be permanent.
	Eyelid skin darkening, which may be reversible, has been reported. Gradual changes to eyelashes and vellus hair around the treated eye include increased length, thickness, pigmentation, number of lashes or hairs, and misdirected growth of eyelashes. Eyelash changes are usually reversible upon discontinuation of treatment.
Adverse Reactions	Eyelash changes (increased length, thickness, pigmentation, and number of lashes); eyelid skin darkening; intraocular

inflammation (iritis/uveitis); iris pigmentation changes; and macular edema, including cystoid macular edema, which have mainly occurred in aphakic patients, in pseudophakic patients with a torn posterior lens capsule, or in patients with known risk factors for macular edema. Should be used with caution in patients who do not have an intact posterior capsule or who have known risk factors for macular edema and in patients with a history of intraocular inflammation (iritis/uveitis); should generally not be used in patients with active intraocular inflammation. There is limited experience in the treatment of angle closure, inflammatory, or neovascular glaucoma.

Controlled clinical trials: Symptoms reported in 5–15% of patients—blurred vision, burning and stinging, conjunctival hyperemia, foreign-body sensation, itching, increased pigmentation of the iris, and punctate epithelial keratopathy. Local conjunctival hyperemia was observed; however, less than 1% of the patients required discontinuation of therapy because of intolerance to conjunctival hyperemia. Symptoms reported in 1–4% of patients—dry eye, excessive tearing, eye pain, lid crusting, lid discomfort/pain, lid edema, lid erythema, photophobia. Symptoms reported in less than 1% of patients—conjunctivitis, diplopia, and discharge. Extremely rare reports—retinal artery embolus, retinal detachment, vitreous hemorrhage from diabetic retinopathy. Most common systemic adverse events—URTI/cold/flu, which occurred at a rate of approximately 4%. Chest pain/angina pectoris, muscle/joint/back pain, and rash/allergic skin reaction each occurred at a rate of 1–2%. *Postmarketing use in clinical practice*: asthma and exacerbation of asthma; corneal edema and erosions; dyspnea; eyelash and vellus hair changes (increased length, thickness, pigmentation, and number); eyelid skin darkening; herpes keratitis; intraocular inflammation (iritis/uveitis); keratitis; macular edema, including cystoid macular edema; misdirected eyelashes, sometimes resulting in eye irritation; toxic epidermal necrolysis.

Pregnancy Category C.

Drug Interactions In vitro studies have shown that precipitation occurs when eye drops containing thimerosal are mixed with Xalatan. If such drugs are used, they should be administered at least 5 min apart.

Leflunomide

Brand Name	Arava.
Class of Drug	Prodrug. When converted to active metabolite, inhibits activated T-cell proliferation; immunomodulatory activity through inhibition of dihydro-orotate dehydrogenase, an enzyme involved in de novo pyrimidine synthesis.
Indications	FDA-approved for rheumatoid arthritis; patients with uveitis intolerant of or unresponsive to methotrexate.
Dosage Form	Oral tablets 10 mg, 20 mg, 100 mg.
Dose	Loading dose of 100 mg/day for 3 days followed by 20 mg/day maintenance (reduced to 10 mg/day if mild hepatotoxicity present).
Contraindications	In patients with a known hypersensitivity to the product or any of its components; patients with liver or renal disease; women who are, or may become, pregnant; patients already immunosuppressed or infected.
Warnings	Pregnancy must be excluded before starting treatment and should be avoided during treatment and prior to depletion of the drug elimination procedure after treatment. Not recommended for patients with severe immunodeficiency; bone marrow dysplasia; or severe, uncontrolled infections.
Adverse Reactions	Hepatotoxicity, leukopenia, gastrointestinal upset, anorexia, rash, alopecia, diarrhea. Monitor CBC with differential, ALT, and AST every 2 weeks for first month then every 4–6 weeks.
Pregnancy Category	X.
Drug Interactions	Safety and efficacy in the pediatric population have not been studied; use in patients younger than 18 years of age is not recommended. Increased side effects may occur when given concomitantly with hepatotoxic substances. Rifampin significantly increases serum levels of leflunomide. Active metabolite (M1) causes increased free-plasma levels of most NSAIDs by inhibiting cytochrome P-450.

Levobunolol Hydrochloride

Brand Name	Betagan.
Class of Drug	Glaucoma. Nonselective beta-adrenergic-blocking agent, equipotent at both beta-1 and beta-2 receptors.
Indications	IOP reduction in patients with chronic OAG or ocular hypertension.
Dosage Form	Topical ophthalmic solution 0.25%, 0.5%.

Dose

Typical dosing with 0.25% ophthalmic solution is 1–2 drops two times per day. In patients with more severe or uncontrolled glaucoma, 0.5% solution can be administered two times per day As with any new medication, careful monitoring of patients is advised. Dosages above 1 drop 0.5% two times per day are not generally more effective. Patients should not typically use two or more topical ophthalmic beta-adrenergic-blocking agents simultaneously.

Contraindications

In patients with bronchial asthma or history of bronchial asthma or severe chronic obstructive pulmonary disease; sinus bradycardia; second- and third-degree AV block; overt cardiac failure; cardiogenic shock; hypersensitivity to the product or any of its components. Should be used with caution in patients with a known hypersensitivity to other beta-adrenoceptor-blocking agents.

Warnings

As with other topically applied ophthalmic drugs, may be absorbed systemically. The same adverse reactions found with systemic administration of beta-adrenergic-blocking agents may occur with topical administration. For example, severe respiratory reactions and cardiac reactions, including death due to bronchospasm in patients with asthma and, rarely, death in association with cardiac failure, have been reported with topical application of beta-adrenergic-blocking agents. *Patients with history cardiac failure*: Beta-adrenergic blockade may precipitate more severe failure. *Patients without history of cardiac failure*: Continued depression of the myocardium with beta-blocking agents over a period of time can, in some cases, lead to cardiac failure. At the first sign or symptom of cardiac failure, discontinue therapy. *Obstructive pulmonary disease*: Patients with chronic obstructive pulmonary disease (e.g., chronic bronchitis, emphysema) of mild or moderate severity, bronchospastic disease, or a history of bronchospastic disease (other than bronchial asthma or a history of bronchial asthma, in which Betagan is contraindicated) should, in general, not receive beta-blockers, including Betagan. However, if Betagan is deemed necessary in such patients, then it should be administered cautiously since it may block bronchodilation produced by endogenous and exogenous catecholamine stimulation of beta-2 receptors. *Major surgery*: The necessity or desirability of withdrawal of beta-adrenergic-blocking agents prior to major surgery is controversial. Beta-adrenergic blockade impairs the ability of the heart to respond to beta-adrenergically mediated reflex stimuli. This may augment the risk of general anesthesia in surgical procedures. Some patients receiving beta-adrenergic-blocking agents have been subject to protracted severe hypotension during anesthesia. Difficulty in restarting and maintaining the heartbeat has also been reported. For these reasons, in patients undergoing elective surgery, gradual withdrawal of beta-adrenergic-blocking agents may be appropriate. If necessary during surgery, the effects of beta-adrenergic-blocking agents may be reversed by sufficient doses of such agonists as isoproterenol, dopamine, dobutamine, or levarterenol. *Diabetes mellitus*: Beta-adrenergic-blocking agents should be administered with caution in patients subject to spontaneous hypoglycemia or to diabetic patients (especially those with labile diabetes) receiving insulin or oral hypoglycemic agents; may mask the signs and symptoms of acute hypoglycemia. *Thyrotoxicosis*: Beta-adrenergic blocking agents may mask certain clinical signs (e.g., tachycardia) of hyperthyroidism. Patients suspected of developing thyrotoxicosis should be managed carefully to avoid abrupt withdrawal of beta-adrenergic-blocking agents, which might precipitate a thyroid storm. These products contain sodium metabisulfite, a sulfite that may cause allergic-type reactions, including anaphylactic symptoms and life-threatening or less-severe asthmatic episodes in certain susceptible people. Overall prevalence of sulfite sensitivity in the general population is unknown and probably low; it is seen more frequently in asthmatic than in nonasthmatic people.

Adverse Reactions Should be used with caution in patients receiving a beta-adrenergic-blocking agent orally because of the potential for additive effects on systemic beta blockade or IOP. Patients should not typically use two or more topical ophthalmic beta-adrenergic-blocking agents simultaneously.*Cardiovascular*: Because of the potential effects on blood pressure and pulse rates, these medications must be used cautiously in patients with cerebrovascular insufficiency. Should signs or symptoms develop that suggest reduced cerebral blood flow while using Betagan ophthalmic solution, alternative therapy should be considered. *Muscle weakness*: Beta-adrenergic blockade has been reported to potentiate muscle weakness consistent with certain myasthenic symptoms (e.g., diplopia, ptosis, and generalized weakness). *Clinical trials*: Has been associated with transient ocular burning and stinging in up to one in three patients, and with blepharoconjunctivitis in up to one in twenty patients. Decreases in heart rate and blood pressure have been reported. *Reported rarely*: iridocyclitis, headache, transient ataxia, dizziness, lethargy, urticaria, pruritus; decreased corneal sensitivity has been noted in a small number of patients; although levobunolol has minimal membrane-stabilizing activity, there remains a possibility of decreased corneal sensitivity after prolonged use. *Other adverse reactions either with Betagan or ophthalmic use of other beta-adrenergic-blocking agents*: Body as a whole—headache, asthenia, chest pain. Cardiovascular—bradycardia, arrhythmia, hypotension, syncope, heart block, cerebral vascular accident, cerebral ischemia, congestive heart failure, palpitation, cardiac arrest. Digestive—nausea, diarrhea. Psychiatric—depression, confusion, increase in signs and symptoms of myasthenia gravis, paresthesia. Skin—hypersensitivity, including localized and generalized rash, alopecia, Stevens–Johnson syndrome. Respiratory—bronchospasm (predominantly in patients with preexisting bronchospastic disease), respiratory failure, dyspnea, nasal congestion. Urogenital—impotence. Endocrine—masked symptoms of hypoglycemia in insulin-dependent diabetics. Special senses—signs and symptoms of keratitis; blepharoptosis; visual disturbances, including refractive changes (due to withdrawal of miotic therapy in some cases); diplopia; ptosis. Other reactions associated with the oral use of nonselective adrenergic receptor blocking agents should be considered potential effects with ophthalmic use of these agents.

Pregnancy Category C.

Drug Interactions Although Betagan used alone has little or no effect on pupil size, mydriasis resulting from concomitant therapy with epinephrine may occur. Close observation is recommended when a beta-blocker is administered to patients receiving catecholamine-depleting drugs, such as reserpine, because of possible additive effects and the production of hypotension and/or marked bradycardia, which may produce vertigo, syncope, or postural hypotension. Patients receiving beta-adrenergic-blocking agents along with either oral or i.v. calcium antagonists should be monitored for possible AV conduction disturbances, left ventricular failure, and hypotension. In patients with impaired cardiac function, simultaneous use should be avoided altogether. Concomitant use of beta-adrenergic-blocking agents with digitalis and calcium antagonists may have additive effects on prolonging AV conduction time. Phenothiazine-related compounds and beta-adrenergic-blocking agents may have additive hypotensive effects due to each inhibiting metabolism of the other.*Risk of anaphylactic reaction*: While taking beta-blockers, patients with a history of severe anaphylactic reaction to a variety of allergens may be more reactive to repeated challenge, either accidental, diagnostic, or therapeutic. Such patients may be unresponsive to the usual doses of epinephrine used to treat allergic reaction.

Levocabastine Hydrochloride

Brand Name   Livostin.
Class of Drug   Selective histamine H_1 antagonist.
Indications   Temporary relief of signs and symptoms of seasonal allergic conjunctivitis.

Dosage Form	Topical ophthalmic suspension 0.05%.
Dose	1 drop to affected eye(s) four times per day.
Contraindications	In patients with a known or suspected hypersensitivity to the product or any of its components. It should not be used while soft contact lenses are being worn.
Warnings	For topical use only.Not for injection.
Adverse Reactions	*Most frequent*: mild, transient stinging and burning (29%) and headache (5%). *Other, reported in approximately 1–3% of patients*: visual disturbances, dry mouth, fatigue, pharyngitis, eye pain/dryness, somnolence, red eyes, lacrimation/discharge, cough, nausea, rash/erythema, eyelid edema, dyspnea.
Pregnancy Category	C.

Levofloxacin

Brand Name	Quixin.
Class of Drug	Fluoroquinolone antibacterial. Inhibition of bacterial topoisomerase IV and DNA gyrase
Indications	For the treatment of bacterial conjunctivitis caused by susceptible strains of the following organisms: Aerobic grampositive—*Corynebacterium* spp.*, *S. aureus*, *S. epidermidis*, *S. pneumoniae*, *Streptococcus* (groups C/F/G), VGS. Aerobic gram-negative—*Acinetobacter lwoffii**, *H. influenzae*, *S. marcescens**. (*Efficacy for this organism was studied in fewer than ten infections.)
Dosage Form	Topical ophthalmic solution 0.5%.
Dose	Days 1 and 2: 1–2 drops to affected eye(s) every 2 h while awake up to eight times per day; days 3–7: 1–2 drops to affected eye(s) every 4 h while awake up to four times per day.
Contraindications	In patients with a history of hypersensitivity to the product or any of its components or to other quinolones.
Warnings	In patients receiving systemic quinolones, serious and occasionally fatal hypersensitivity (anaphylactic) reactions have been reported, some following the first dose. Some reactions were accompanied by cardiovascular collapse, loss of consciousness, angioedema (including laryngeal, pharyngeal, or facial edema), airway obstruction, dyspnea, urticaria, and itching. If an allergic reaction occurs, discontinue the drug. Serious acute hypersensitivity reactions may require immediate emergency treatment. Oxygen and airway management should be administered as clinically indicated. Should not be injected subconjunctivally, nor should it be introduced directly into the anterior chamber of the eye.
Adverse Reactions	*Systemic*: quinolones have been associated with hypersensitivity reactions, even following a single dose. Discontinue use

immediately and contact your physician at the first sign of a rash or allergic reaction. *Most frequently reported* in the overall study population were transient decreased vision, fever, foreign-body sensation, headache, transient ocular burning, ocular pain or discomfort, pharyngitis, and photophobia (approximately 1–3% of patients). *Others*: include allergic reactions, lid edema, ocular dryness, and ocular itching (less than 1% of patients).

Pregnancy Category C.

Drug Interactions Specific drug interaction studies have not been conducted. However, systemic administration of some quinolones has been shown to elevate plasma concentrations of theophylline, interfere with the metabolism of caffeine, enhance the effects of the oral anticoagulant warfarin and its derivatives, and has been associated with transient elevations in serum creatinine in patients receiving systemic cyclosporine concomitantly.

Lidocaine

Brand Name	Xylocaine.
Class of Drug	Local anesthetic.
Indications	Local anesthesia.
Dosage Form	Parenteral for injection (0.5/½%) maximum dose 200 mg.
Dose	Maximum 2.9 mg/kg body weight. Rapid onset (<2 min), last for 1–1.5 h; in combination with vasoconstrictor, up to 4 h.
Contraindications	*Most significant*: Adams–Stokes syndrome, lidocaine toxicity, severe heart block. *Significant*: congestive heart failure, hypovolemia, incomplete AV heart block, reduced hepatic blood flow, shock, sinus bradycardia, Wolff–Parkinson–White pattern. *Possibly significant*: renal disease.
Adverse Reactions	Allergic reactions, anaphylaxis, CNS toxicity, erythema, methemoglobinemia, myocardial, dysfunction, nausea, pruritus, skin rash, sneezing, urticaria, vasodilation of blood vessels, vomiting.
Drug Interactions	Possibly safe in pregnancy. It is not known whether this drug or its metabolites are excreted in human milk. Relative contraindication:<u>risk of systemic toxicity possible in pediatric patients</u>.
Pregnancy Category	B.

Lodoxamide Tromethamine

Brand Name	Alomide.
Class of Drug	Mast cell stabilizer.
Indications	Ocular disorders referred to as vernal keratoconjunctivitis, vernal conjunctivitis, and vernal keratitis.*Off-label*: treatment of seasonal allergic conjunctivitis.
Dosage Form	Topical ophthalmic solution 0.1%.
Dose	Adults, and children older than 2 years of age: 1–2 drops to affected eye(s) four times per day for up to 3 months.
Contraindications	In patients with hypersensitivity to the product or any of its components.
Warnings	<u>Not for injection.</u>
Adverse Reactions	*Ocular*: During clinical studies, the most frequently reported were transient burning, stinging, or discomfort upon instillation, which occurred in approximately 15% of the subjects. Other events occurring in 1–5% of subjects included ocular itching/pruritus, blurred vision, dry eye, tearing/discharge, hyperemia, crystalline deposits, and foreign body sensation. Events that occurred in less than 1% of subjects included corneal erosion/ulcer, scales on lid/lash, eye pain, ocular edema/swelling, ocular warming sensation, ocular fatigue, chemosis, corneal abrasion, anterior chamber cells, keratopathy/keratitis, blepharitis, allergy, sticky sensation, and epitheliopathy. *Nonocular*: headache (1.5%) and (at less than 1%) heat sensation, dizziness, somnolence, nausea, stomach discomfort, sneezing, dry nose, and rash.
Pregnancy Category	B.

Loteprednol Etabonate

Brand Name	Alrex.
Class of Drug	Corticosteroid.
Indications	For the temporary relief of the signs and symptoms of seasonal allergic conjunctivitis.
Dosage Form	Topical ophthalmic suspension 0.2%.
Dose	1 drop to affected eye(s) four times per day.
Contraindications	As with other ophthalmic corticosteroids, in most viral diseases of the cornea and conjunctiva, including epithelial herpes simplex keratitis (dendritic keratitis), vaccinia, and varicella; also in mycobacterial infection of the eye and fungal diseases of ocular structures. In patients with a known or

suspected hypersensitivity to the product or any of its components or to other corticosteroids.

Warnings

Prolonged use of corticosteroids may result in glaucoma with damage to the optic nerve, defects in visual acuity and fields of vision, and posterior subcapsular cataract formation. Steroids should be used with caution in the presence of glaucoma. Prolonged use of corticosteroids may suppress the host response and thus increase the hazard of secondary ocular infections. In those diseases causing thinning of the cornea or sclera, perforations have been known to occur with the use of topical steroids. In acute purulent conditions of the eye, steroids may mask infection or enhance existing infection. Use of ocular steroids may prolong the course and may exacerbate the severity of many viral infections of the eye (including herpes simplex). Employment of corticosteroid medication in the treatment of patients with a history of herpes simplex requires great caution. If signs and symptoms fail to improve after 2 days, the patient should be re-evaluated. If this product is used for 10 days or longer, IOP should be monitored. Fungus invasion must be considered in any persistent corneal ulceration where a steroid has been used or is in use. Fungal cultures should be taken when appropriate.

Adverse Reactions

Reactions associated with ophthalmic steroids include elevated IOP, which may be associated with optic nerve damage; visual acuity and field defects; posterior subcapsular cataract formation; secondary ocular infection from pathogens, including herpes simplex; and perforation of the globe where there is thinning of the cornea or sclera. *Ocular*: in clinical studies, included abnormal vision/blurring, burning on instillation, chemosis, discharge, dry eyes, epiphora, foreign-body sensation, itching, injection, and photophobia (in 5–15% of patients); included conjunctivitis, corneal abnormalities, eyelid erythema, keratoconjunctivitis, ocular irritation/pain/discomfort, papillae, and uveitis (in less than 5% of patients); some of these events were similar to the underlying ocular disease being studied. *Nonocular*: included headache, rhinitis, and pharyngitis (in less than 15% of patients).

In a summation of controlled, randomized studies of individuals treated for 28 days or longer with loteprednol etabonate, the incidence of significant elevation of IOP ($\geq$10 mmHg) was 2% (15/901) among patients receiving loteprednol etabonate, 7% (11/164) among patients receiving 1% prednisolone acetate, and 0.5% (3/583) among patients receiving placebo. Among a smaller study group of patients treated with Alrex, the incidence of clinically significant increases in IOP ($\geq$10 mmHg) was 1% (1/133) with Alrex and 1% (1/135) with placebo.

Pregnancy Category

C.

Brand Name

Lotemax.

Class of Drug

Corticosteroid.

Indications   For the treatment of steroid responsive inflammatory con-
                              ditions of the palpebral and bulbar conjunctiva, cornea, and
                              anterior segment of the globe, such as allergic conjunctivitis,
                              acne rosacea, superficial punctate keratitis, herpes zoster ke-
                              ratitis, iritis, cyclitis, selected infective conjunctivitides, when
                              the inherent hazard of steroid use is accepted in order to
                              obtain an advisable diminution in edema and inflammation.
                              Less effective than prednisolone acetate 1% in two 28-day
                              controlled clinical studies in acute anterior uveitis. Also indi-
                              cated for postoperative inflammation following ocular surge-
                              ry.
Dosage Form   Topical ophthalmic suspension 0.5%.
Dose   Shake vigorously before using. *Steroid-responsive disease
                              treatment*: 1–2 drops into the conjunctival sac of affected
                              eye(s) four times per day. During initial treatment within the
                              first week, the dosing may be increased up to 1 drop every
                              hour, if necessary. Care should be taken not to discontinue
                              therapy prematurely. If signs and symptoms fail to improve
                              after 2 days, the patient should be re-evaluated. *Postoperative
                              inflammation*: 1–2 drops into the conjunctival sac of operated
                              eye(s) four times per day beginning 24 h after surgery and
                              continuing throughout the first 2 weeks of the postoperative
                              period.
Contraindications   As with other ophthalmic corticosteroids, in most viral di-
                              seases of the cornea and conjunctiva, including epithelial
                              herpes simplex keratitis (dendritic keratitis), vaccinia, and
                              varicella; also in mycobacterial infection of the eye and fun-
                              gal diseases of ocular structures. In patients with a known
                              or suspected hypersensitivity to the product or any of its
                              components or to other corticosteroids. Should not be used
                              in patients who require a more potent corticosteroid for this
                              indication.
Warnings   See »Alrex.«
Adverse Reactions   See »Alrex.«
Pregnancy Category   C.

Mannitol

Brand Name Osmitrol.

Class of Drug Nonelectrolyte osmotic diuretic.

Indications Reduction of elevated IOP when the pressure cannot be lowered by other means.

Dosage Form Solution for i.v. injection: 5%, 10%, 15%, 20%, 25%.

Dose For reduction of IOP: 1.5–2 g/kg as a 20% solution (7.5–10 ml/kg) or as a 15% solution (10–13 ml/g) over a period of as short as 30 min. When used preoperatively, administer 1–1.5 h before surgery to achieve maximum effect. Total dosage, concentration, and rate of administration should be governed by the nature and severity of the condition being treated, fluid requirement, and urinary output. Usual adult dosage ranges from 50 g to 200 g in a 24-h period, but in most cases, an adequate response will be achieved at a dosage of approximately 100 g/24 h. Rate of administration is usually adjusted to maintain a urine flow of at least 30–50 ml/hr. This outline of dosage and administration is only a general guide.

Contraindications In patients with well-established anuria due to severe renal disease; severe pulmonary congestion or frank pulmonary edema; active intracranial bleeding except during craniotomy; severe dehydration; progressive renal damage or dysfunction after institution of mannitol therapy, including increasing oliguria and azotemia; progressive heart failure or pulmonary congestion after institution of therapy.

Warnings May obscure and intensify inadequate hydration or hypovolemia by sustaining diuresis. Electrolyte measurements, including sodium and potassium, are important in monitoring infusion. Carefully evaluate cardiovascular status before rapid administration because sudden expansion of the extracellular fluid may lead to fulminating congestive heart failure (CHF). A test dose should be utilized in patients with severe impairment of renal function; a second test dose may be tried if there is an inadequate response, but no more than two test doses should be attempted. If urine output continues to decline during infusion, the patient's clinical status should be closely reviewed and infusion suspended if necessary. Osmotic nephrosis, a reversible vacuolization of the tubules of no known clinical significance, may proceed to severe, irreversible nephrosis requiring close monitoring during infusion. Electrolyte-free mannitol solutions should not be given simultaneously with blood. If blood is given simultaneously, add at least 20 mEq of sodium chloride to each liter of mannitol solution to avoid pseudoagglutination.

Adverse Reactions Reactions that may occur because of the solution or the technique of administration include febrile response, infection at the site of injection, venous thrombosis or phlebitis extending from the site of injection, extravasation, and hypervolemia. Isolated cases, such as pulmonary congestion, fluid and electrolyte imbalance, acidosis, electrolyte loss, dryness of mouth, thirst, marked diuresis, urinary retention, edema, headache, blurred vision, convulsions, nausea, vomiting, rhinitis, arm pain, skin necrosis, thrombophlebitis, chills, dizziness, urticaria, dehydration, hypotension, tachycardia, fever, and angina-like chest pains have been reported during or following infusion. Too rapid infusion of hypertonic solutions may cause local pain and venous irritation. Rate of administration should be adjusted according to tolerance. Use of the largest peripheral vein and a small bore needle is recommended. The physician should also be alert to the possibility of adverse reactions to drug additives. Prescribing information for drug additives to be administered in this manner should be consulted. If an adverse reaction does occur, discontinue the infusion, evaluate the patient, institute appropriate therapeutic countermeasures, and save the remainder of the fluid for examination if deemed necessary.

Pregnancy Category   C.

Medrysone

Brand Name   HMS.
Class of Drug   Synthetic corticosteroid with topical anti-inflammatory activity.
Indications   For the treatment of allergic conjunctivitis, vernal conjunctivitis, episcleritis, and epinephrine sensitivity.
Dosage Form   Topical ophthalmic suspension 1%.
Dose   1 drop in the conjunctival sac up to every 4 h.
Contraindications   In most viral diseases of the cornea and conjunctiva, including epithelial herpes simplex keratitis (dendritic keratitis), vaccinia, and varicella; also mycobacterial infection of the eye and fungal diseases of ocular structures; in patients with a known or suspected hypersensitivity to the product or any of its components or to other corticosteroids.
Warnings   Not recommended for use in iritis and uveitis as therapeutic effectiveness has not been demonstrated in these conditions. Prolonged use of corticosteroids may result in glaucoma with damage to the optic nerve, defects in visual acuity and fields of vision, and posterior subcapsular cataract formation. Prolonged use may also suppress the host immune response and thus increase the hazard of secondary ocular infections. Prolonged use of corticosteroids may result in glaucoma with damage to the optic

nerve, defects in visual acuity and fields of vision, posterior subcapsular cataract formation, and may also suppress the host immune response and thus increase the hazard of secondary ocular infections. Various ocular diseases and long-term use of topical corticosteroids have been known to cause corneal and scleral thinning. Use of topical corticosteroids in the presence of thin corneal or scleral tissue may lead to perforation. Acute purulent infections of the eye may be masked or activity enhanced by the presence of corticosteroid medication. If this product is used for 10 days or longer, IOP should be routinely monitored even though it may be difficult in children and uncooperative patients. Steroids should be used with caution in the presence of glaucoma and IOP should be checked frequently. Use of steroids after cataract surgery may delay healing, increase the incidence of bleb formation, prolong the course and may exacerbate the severity of many viral infections of the eye (including herpes simplex). Employment of corticosteroid medication in the treatment of patients with a history of herpes simplex requires great caution; frequent slit lamp microscopy is recommended. Corticosteroids are not effective in mustard gas keratitis and Sjögren's keratoconjunctivitis.

Adverse Reactions If signs and symptoms fail to improve after 2 days, the patient should be re-evaluated. As fungal infections of the cornea are particularly prone to develop coincidentally with long-term local corticosteroid applications, fungal invasion should be suspected in any persistent corneal ulceration where a corticosteroid has been used or is in use. Fungal cultures should be taken when appropriate. Adverse reactions include, in decreasing order of frequency, elevation of IOP with possible development of glaucoma and infrequent optic nerve damage, posterior subcapsular cataract formation, delayed wound healing. Although systemic effects are extremely uncommon, there have been rare occurrences of systemic hypercorticoidism after use of topical steroids. Corticosteroid-containing preparations have also been reported to cause acute anterior uveitis and perforation of the globe. Keratitis, conjunctivitis, corneal ulcers, mydriasis, conjunctival hyperemia, loss of accommodation, and ptosis have occasionally been reported following local use of corticosteroids. Development of secondary ocular infection (bacterial, fungal, and viral) has occurred. Fungal and viral infections of the cornea are particularly prone to develop coincidentally with long-term application of steroids. The possibility of fugal invasion should be considered in any persistent corneal ulceration where steroid treatment has been used. Transient burning and stinging upon instillation and other minor symptoms of ocular irritation have been reported with the use of HMS suspension; other adverse events reported include allergic reactions, foreign-body sensation, and visual disturbance (blurry vision).

Pregnancy Category   C.

Mepivacaine

Brand Name	Carbocaine; Isocaine; Polocaine.
Class of Drug	Local anesthetic.
Indications	Local anesthesia.
Dosage Form	Parenteral for injection (0.5/1/2%). Maximum dose 300 mg.
Dose	Maximum dose 4 mg/kg body weight. Rapid onset (<2 min), lasts for 1.5–3 h.
Contraindications	*Most significant*: infection at site. *Significant*: disease of cardiovascular system, myasthenia gravis, plasma, cholinesterase deficiency. *Possibly significant*: liver disease, renal disease.
Warnings	Local anesthetics should only be employed by clinicians who are well versed in diagnosis and management of dose-related toxicity and other acute emergencies that might arise from the block to be employed, and then only after ensuring the immediate availability of oxygen, other resuscitative drugs, cardiopulmonary resuscitation equipment, and the personnel resources needed for proper management of toxic reactions and related emergencies.
Adverse Reactions	Allergic reactions, anaphylaxis, CNS toxicity, erythema, methemoglobinemia, myocardial, dysfunction, nausea, pruritus, skin rash, sneezing, urticaria, vasodilation of blood vessels, vomiting.
Pregnancy Category	C.
Drug Interactions	Only when necessary in pregnancy. It is not known whether this drug or its metabolites are excreted in human milk. *Relative contraindication*: <u>risk of systemic toxicity possible in pediatric patients</u>.

Methazolamide

Brand Name	Neptazane; GlaucTabs; MZM.
Class of Drug	CAI (sulfonamide).
Indications	In the treatment of ocular conditions where lowering IOP is likely to be of therapeutic benefit, such as chronic OAG, se-

condary glaucoma, and preoperatively in acute ACG where lowering IOP is desired before surgery.

Dosage Form   Oral tablets 25 mg, 50 mg.

Dose   Effective therapeutic dose varies from 50 mg to 100 mg two to three times per day. May be used concomitantly with miotic and osmotic agents.

Contraindications   In situations in which sodium and/or potassium serum levels are depressed, in cases of marked kidney or liver disease or dysfunction, in adrenal gland failure, and in hyperchloremic acidosis. In patients with cirrhosis, use may precipitate the development of hepatic encephalopathy. Long-term administration is contraindicated in patients with ACG since organic closure of the angle may occur in spite of lowered IOP.

Warnings   Fatalities have occurred, although rarely, due to severe reactions to sulfonamides, including Stevens–Johnson syndrome, toxic epidermal necrolysis, fulminant hepatic necrosis, agranulocytosis, aplastic anemia, and other blood dyscrasias. Hypersensitivity reactions may recur when a sulfonamide is readministered, irrespective of the route of administration. If hypersensitivity or other serious reactions occur, use of this drug should be discontinued. Caution is advised for patients receiving high-dose aspirin and methazolamide concomitantly, as anorexia, tachypnea, lethargy, coma, and death have been reported with concomitant use of high-dose aspirin and carbonic anhydrase inhibitors. Potassium excretion is increased initially upon administration. In patients with cirrhosis or hepatic insufficiency, could precipitate a hepatic coma. In patients with pulmonary obstruction or emphysema, where alveolar ventilation may be impaired, should be used with caution because it may precipitate or aggravate acidosis.

Adverse Reactions   *Most often early in therapy*: include paresthesias, particularly a »tingling« feeling in the extremities; hearing dysfunction or tinnitus; fatigue; malaise; loss of appetite; taste alteration; gastrointestinal disturbances, such as nausea, vomiting, and diarrhea; polyuria; and occasional instances of drowsiness and confusion. Metabolic acidosis and electrolyte imbalance may occur. Transient myopia has been reported; invariably subsides upon diminution or discontinuance of the medication. *Other occasional*: include urticaria, melena, hematuria, glycosuria, hepatic insufficiency, flaccid paralysis, photosensitivity, convulsions, and, rarely, crystalluria and renal calculi. *Fatalities*: have occurred, although rarely, due to severe reactions to sulfonamides, including Stevens–Johnson syndrome, toxic epidermal necrolysis, fulminate hepatic necrosis, agranulocytosis, aplastic anemia, and other blood dyscrasias.

Pregnancy Category   C.

Drug Interactions   Should be used with caution in patients on steroid therapy because of the potential for developing hypokalemia. Caution is advised for patients receiving high-dose aspirin concomitantly, as anorexia, tachypnea, lethargy, coma, and death have been reported with concomitant use of high-dose aspirin and CAI.

Methotrexate

Brand Name   Rheumatrex; Folex; Mexate.

Class of Drug   Antimetabolite. Folic acid antagonist; prevents conversion of dihydrofolate to tetrahydrofolate; inhibits DNA replication and RNA transcription.

Indications   Agent of choice in maintenance therapy of acute lymphocytic leukemia; effective in treatment of a variety of systemic inflammatory conditions, including psoriasis, rheumatoid arthritis, JRA, Reiter's disease, polymyositis, sarcoidosis, ankylosing spondylitis, and inflammatory bowel disease.*Ophthalmic*: steroid-resistant cyclitis; sympathetic ophthalmia recalcitrant to conventional therapy; steroid-resistant uveitis; pediatric uveitis refractory to more conventional therapy; scleritis associated with collagen vascular diseases, such as Reiter's syndrome and rheumatoid arthritis; chronic uveitis-vitreitis; retinal vasculitis; inflammatory pseudotumor; orbital myositis; scleritis; sarcoid-associated panuveitis.

Dosage Form   Rheumatrex:*Oral*—2.5 mg tablets. Folex; Mexate: *Solution for injection*: 2.5, 25 mg/ml. *Powder*: 20 mg, 50 mg, 100 mg, 250 mg, 1 g vials. *Folex (Adria) solution*: 25 mg/ml.

Dose   Weekly dose of 2.5–10 mg orally, i.m., or i.v. in a 36–48 h period to a maximum of 50 mg/week. Close monitoring of LFTs at baseline and at 4- to 8-week intervals; elevation of LFTs to twice normal requires discontinuation or reduction. Monitor CBC; treatment should be stopped if there is a significant drop in blood counts.

Contraindications   In pregnant or nursing women; patients with know alcoholism, alcoholic liver disease, or chronic liver disease of any etiology; patients with immunodeficiency states, preexisting blood dyscrasias, or bone marrow suppression; any patient with a known hypersensitivity the product or any of its components. Not recommended for women of childbearing potential unless there is clear medical evidence that the benefits can be expected to outweigh the considered risks.

Warnings   Reported to cause fetal death and/or congenital anomalies. Unexpectedly severe (sometimes fatal) bone marrow suppression, aplastic anemia, and gastrointestinal toxicity have been reported with concomitant administration of methotrexate (usually in high dosage) with some NSAIDs. Elimination is reduced in patients with impaired renal function, ascites, or pleural effusions. Causes hepatotoxicity, fibrosis, and cirrhosis, but generally only after prolonged use. Acutely, liver enzyme elevations are frequently seen; periodic liver biopsies are usually recommended for psoriatic patients who are under long-term treatment; persistent abnormalities in LFTs may precede appearance of fibrosis or cirrhosis in the rheumatoid arthritis population. Use extreme caution in administering to the elderly with decreased renal and hepatic reserves. Methotrexate-induced lung disease is a potentially dangerous lesion, which may occur acutely at any time at doses as low as 7.5 mg/week and is not always fully reversible. Pulmonary symptoms (especially a dry, nonproductive cough) may require interruption of treatment and careful investigation. Diarrhea and ulcerative stomatitis require interruption of therapy; otherwise, hemorrhagic enteritis and death from intestinal perforation may occur.

Adverse Reactions *Hematologic*: myelosuppression, leucopenia (WBC less than 3,000/mm^3), aplastic anemia, thrombocytopenia (platelet count less than 100,000/mm^3), pancytopenia with low dose therapy. *GI*: nausea, ulcerative mucositis, stomatitis, diarrhea, all of which may respond to dosage reduction. *Hepatotoxicity*: acute elevation of transaminases; usually reversible. Chronic hepatotoxicity (fibrosis and cirrhosis) may potentially be fatal; generally has occurred after prolonged use (generally 2 years or more) and after a total dose of at least 1.5 g; appeared to be a function of total cumulative dose and to be enhanced by alcoholism, obesity, diabetes, and advanced age. *Pulmonary*: acute pneumonitis, pulmonary fibrosis, interstitial pneumonitis, dyspnea, coughing, exercise intolerance. Potentially fatal opportunistic infections, especially *P. carinii* pneumonia, may occur. *Dermatologic*: rash, pruritus, dermatitis, alopecia, erythematous rashes, urticaria, photosensitivity, pigmentary changes, ecchymosis, telangiectasia, acne, furunculosis, erythema multiforme, toxic epidermal necrolysis, Stevens–Johnson syndrome, skin necrosis, skin ulceration, and exfoliative. *Other*: pancreatitis, acute renal failure with high-dose regimens, oligospermia, and dizziness. *Ocular*: include irritation, photophobia, aggravation of seborrheic blepharitis, and epiphora.

Pregnancy Category X.

Drug Interactions Potential serious adverse reactions in breast-feeding infants. Published clinical studies evaluating use in children and adolescents (i.e., patients 2–16 years of age) with JRA demonstrated safety comparable to that observed in adults with rheumatoid arthritis. Oral antibiotics, such as tetracycline, chloramphenicol, and nonabsorbable broad spectrum antibiotics, may decrease intestinal absorption of methotrexate or interfere with the enterohepatic circulation by inhibiting bowel flora and suppressing metabolism of the drug by bacteria. Treatment with drugs such as NSAIDs or probenecid impairs renal blood flow or tubular secretion, may delay drug excretion, and may lead to severe toxicity. Partially bound to serum albumin, and toxicity may be increased because of displacement by certain drugs, such as salicylates, phenylbutazone, phenytoin, and sulfonamides. Renal tubular transport is also diminished by probenecid; use of methotrexate with this drug should be carefully monitored.

Methylcellulose

Brand Name	Murocel.
Class of Drug	Lubricant eye drops.
Indications	See »Hydroxypropyl Methylcellulose.« (Methylcellulose derivatives are also used as wetting agents in more viscous gas permeable contact lens solution.)
Dosage Form	Topical ophthalmic solution 1%.
Dose	See » Hydroxypropyl Methylcellulose.«
Contraindications	See » Hydroxypropyl Methylcellulose.«
Warnings	See »Hydroxypropyl Methylcellulose.«
Adverse Reactions	See »Hydroxypropyl Methylcellulose.«
Drug Interactions	See »Hydroxypropyl Methylcellulose.«

Methylene Blue

Brand Name	Urolene Blue.
Class of Drug	Diagnostic aid, tissue dye.
Indications	To stain tissue before or during ophthalmic surgery or procedure. Methylene blue (methylthionine chloride) exists as dark green crystals. Soluble in water and in chloroform; sparingly soluble in alcohol.
Dosage Form	Injection 10 mg/ml.
Dose	Possesses weak antiseptic properties. Is well absorbed by the gastrointestinal tract and rapidly reduced to leukomethylene blue, which is stabilized in some combination form in the urine; 75% is excreted unchanged.
Contraindications	In patients with a know hypersensitivity to this product or any of its components.
Warnings	Patients should be advised that the urine and/or stools may become blue to blue-green as a result of the excretion of methylene blue.

Adverse Reactions May cause anemia or make methemoglobinemia worse in glucose-6-phosphate dehydrogenase (G6PD) deficiency. In patients with kidney disease, may accumulate in the body. May make cyanide toxicity worse by increasing the amount of cyanide in the blood. Studies on effects in pregnancy have not been done in either humans or animals.

Metipranolol

Brand Name OptiPranolol.

Class of Drug Beta-1 and beta-2 nonselective adrenergic receptor blocker.

Indications Treatment of elevated IOP in patients with ocular hypertension or OAG.

Dosage Form Topical ophthalmic solution 0.3%.

Dose 1 drop two times per day.

Contraindications In patients with bronchial asthma or a history of bronchial asthma or severe chronic obstructive pulmonary disease, symptomatic sinus bradycardia, greater than a first-degree AV block, cardiogenic shock, overt cardiac failure, or hypersensitivity to the product or any of its components.

Warnings As with other topically applied ophthalmic drugs, this drug may be absorbed systemically. Thus, the same adverse reactions found with systemic administration of beta-adrenergic-blocking agents may occur with topical administration. For example, severe respiratory and cardiac reactions, including death due to bronchospasm in patients with asthma, and, rarely, death in association with cardiac failure, have been reported following topical application of beta-adrenergic-blocking agents. Since metipranolol had a minor effect on heart rate and blood pressure in clinical studies, caution should be observed in treating patients with a history of cardiac failure. Treatment should be discontinued at the first evidence of cardiac failure. Metipranolol, or other beta-blockers, should not, in general, be administered to patients with chronic obstructive pulmonary disease (e.g., chronic bronchitis, emphysema) of mild or moderate severity. However, if the drug is necessary such patients, then it should be administered with caution since it may block bronchodilation produced by endogenous and exogenous catecholamine stimulation of beta-2, receptors. Use with caution in patients with cerebrovascular insufficiency. If signs or symptoms suggesting reduced cerebral blood flow develop following initiation of therapy, alternative therapy should be considered.

Adverse Reactions *Clinical trials*: associated with transient local discomfort. *Other ocular*: conjunctivitis, eyelid dermatitis, blepharitis, blurred vision, tearing, brow ache, abnormal vision, photophobia, and edema have been reported in a small number of patients either in U.S. clinical trials or from postmarketing experience in Europe. *Other systemic*: allergic reaction, headache, asthenia, hypertension, myocardial infarct, atrial fibrillation, angina, palpitation bradycardia nausea, rhinitis, dyspnea, epistaxis, bronchitis, coughing, dizziness, anxiety, depression, somnolence, nervousness, arthritis, myalgia, and rash have also been reported in a small number of patients.

Some authorities recommend gradual withdrawal of beta-adrenergic-blocking agents in patients undergoing elective surgery. If necessary during surgery, the effects of beta-adrenergic-blocking agents may be reversed by sufficient doses of such agonists as isoproterenol, dopamine, dobutamine, or levarterenol. While metipranolol has demonstrated a low potential for systemic effect, it should be used with caution in patients with diabetes (especially labile diabetes) because of possible masking of signs and symptoms of acute hypoglycemia. Beta-adrenergic-blocking agents may mask certain signs and symptoms of hyperthyroidism, and their abrupt withdrawal might precipitate a thyroid storm. Beta-adrenergic blockade has been reported to potentiate muscle weakness consistent with certain myasthenic symptoms (e.g., diplopia, ptosis, and generalized weakness). While taking beta-blockers, patients with a history of severe anaphylactic reaction to a variety of allergens may be more reactive to repeated challenge either accidental, diagnostic, or therapeutic. Such patients may be unresponsive to the usual doses of epinephrine used to treat allergic reaction.

Pregnancy Category C.

Drug Interactions Should be used with caution in patients receiving a beta-adrenergic-blocking agent orally because of the potential for additive effects on systemic beta blockade. Close observation is recommended when a beta-blocker is administered to patients receiving catecholamine-depleting drugs, such as reserpine, because of possible additive effects and the production of hypotension and/or bradycardia. Caution should be used in the coadministration of beta-adrenergic-blocking agents, such as metipranolol, and oral or i.v. calcium-channel antagonists because of possible precipitation of left ventricular failure and hypotension. In patients with impaired cardiac function receiving calcium channel antagonists, coadministration should be avoided. The concomitant use of beta-adrenergic-blocking agents with digitalis and calcium-channel antagonists may have additive effects, prolonging AV conduction time. Caution should be used in patients using concomitant adrenergic psychotropic drugs.

Mineral Oil

Brand Name	Refresh P.M.; Duolube; Duratears; Tears Renewed Ointment.
Class of Drug	Eye lubricant ointment. Preservative free.
Indications	Eye lubricant.
Dosage Form	Mineral oil and white petrolatum.
Dose	Apply small amount (approximately 0.6 cm; ¼ in.) of ointment to the inside of the lower eye lid.

Mitomycin

Brand Name	Mutamycin.
Class of Drug	Antineoplastic. Alkylating agent by inhibiting DNA synthesis.
Indications	Off-label: adjuvant in glaucoma surgery, ocular surface, squamous dysplasia, postoperative after pterygium surgery.
Dosage Form	Each vial contains 5 mg, 20 mg, or 40 mg mitomycin. Reconstitute with sterile water to desired concentration; stable for 14 days refrigerated or 7 days at room temperature.
Dose	Concentration of 0.2–0.4 mg/ml soaked in sponge; applied to ocular surface for 1–5 min and then thoroughly irrigated.
Contraindications	In patients who have demonstrated hypersensitive or idiosyncratic reaction to the product or any of its components.
Warnings	Handle and discard in accordance with hospital policies regarding safe use of antineoplastics.
Adverse Reactions	Conjunctival wound leaks, corneal epithelial defects, hypotony associated with permanent reduced visual acuity, serious corneal infections in eyes with preexisting corneal edema increased susceptibility to late-onset bleb infections.*More serious*: corneal melts, scleral ulceration and calcification.
Pregnancy Category	D.
Drug Interactions	Teratological changes have been noted in animal studies. Safety and effectiveness in pediatric patients have not been established.

Moxifloxacin Hydrochloride

Brand Name   Vigamox.
Class of Drug   Fluoroquinolone antibacterial. Inhibition of topoisomerase II
                        (DNA gyrase) and topoisomerase IV.
Indications   For the treatment of bacterial conjunctivitis caused by sus-
                        ceptible strains of the following organisms: Aerobic gram-po-
                        sitive—*Corynebacterium* spp*, *Micrococcus luteus*, *S. aureus*,
                        S. epidermidis, *Staphylococcus hemolyticus*, *Staphylococcus
                        hominis*, *Staphylococcus warneri**, *S. pneumoniae*, *S. viridans*.
                        Aerobic gram-negative—*A. lwoffii**, *H. influenzae*, *H. parain-
                        fluenzae**. Other microorganisms—*C. trachomatis*. (*Efficacy
                        for this organism was studied in fewer than ten infections.)
Dosage Form   Topical ophthalmic solution 0.5%.
Dose   1 drop three times per day for 7 days.
Contraindications   In patients with a history of hypersensitivity the product or
                        any of its components or to other quinolones.
Warnings   Should not be injected subconjunctivally nor introduced di-
                        rectly into anterior chamber. Systemic use has been associa-
                        ted with serious and occasionally fatal anaphylactic reactions.
Adverse Reactions   *Ocular*: conjunctivitis, decreased visual acuity, dry eye, keratitis,
                        ocular discomfort, ocular hyperemia, ocular pain, ocular pruri-
                        tus, subconjunctival hemorrhage, tearing. Occurred in 1–6% of
                        patients. *Nonocular*: included fever, increased cough, infection,
                        otitis media, pharyngitis, rash, rhinitis. Reported in 1–4% of pa-
                        tients.
Pregnancy Category C.
Drug Interactions   In vitro studies indicate that moxifloxacin does not inhibit
                        CYP3A4, CYP2D6, CYP2C9, CYP2C19, or CYP1A2, indicating it
                        is unlikely to alter the pharmacokinetics of drugs metaboli-
                        zed by these cytochrome P-450 isozymes.

Mycophenolate Mofetil

Brand Name   CellCept.
Class of Drug   Prodrug. Metabolized to the active immunosuppressive moi-
                        ety mycophenolate acid. Mycophenolate acid inhibits B- and
                        T-cell proliferation by selective inhibition of inosine mono-
                        phosphate dehydrogenase thus inhibiting de novo purine
                        synthesis and decreasing guanine and DNA synthesis.
Indications   For prevention of solid organ transplant rejection. *Off-label*:
                        treating patients with noninfectious autoimmune inflamma-
                        tory eye disease (scleritis, uveitis).

Dosage Form	*Oral capsules*: 250 mg. *Oral tablets*: 500 mg, *Oral suspension*: 200 mg/ml. *Sterile solution for i.v. injection*: 500 mg/20 ml.
Dose	1,000–2,000 mg/day. Based on pharmacokinetic and safety data in pediatric patients after renal transplantation, the recommended dose of oral suspension is 600 mg/m^2 two times per day (up to maximum of 1 g two times per day).
Contraindications	In patients with hypersensitivity the product or any of its components; i.v. solution in patients allergic to polysorbate 80 (TWEEN); patients immunocompromised before mycophenolate mofetil therapy and those with renal impairment.
Warnings	Increased susceptibility to infection and possible development of lymphoma may result from immunosuppression. Lymphoproliferative disease or lymphoma developed in 0.4–1% of patients receiving mycophenolate mofetil (2 g or 3 g) with other immunosuppressive agents in controlled clinical trials of renal, cardiac, and hepatic transplant patients.
Adverse Reactions	Secondary malignancy, bone marrow suppression, gastrointestinal upset (very common), opportunistic infections, renal and liver toxicity, impotence, anorexia, alopecia, nausea, leukopenia. Monitor CBC with differential, ALT, and AST every 2 weeks for first month then every 4–6 weeks.
Pregnancy Category	C.
Drug Interactions	Adverse effects on fetal development (including malformations) occurred when pregnant rats and rabbits were dosed during organogenesis. These responses occurred at doses lower than those associated with maternal toxicity and at doses below the recommended clinical dose for renal, cardiac, or hepatic transplantation. There are no adequate and well-controlled studies in pregnant women.*Drug interaction*: acyclovir (increased availability of both drugs), antacids (decrease absorption of mycophenolate mofetil), cholestyramine (interfere with enterohepatic circulation and decrease availability of mycophenolate mofetil), cyclosporine (no effect), ganciclovir (increase availability of both, especially in the presence of renal impairment), oral contraceptives (may interfere with availability; consider other methods of contraception).

Naphazoline Hydrochloride

Brand Name   Albalon; Naphcon-A; Vasocon-A; Visine-A; AK-Con; All Clear; All Clear AR; Clear Eyes; Clear Eyes ACR; Opcon-A.

Class of Drug   Sympathomimetic, vasoconstrictor.

Indications   Temporary relief of minor symptoms of ocular pruritus and conjunctival congestion.

Dosage Form   Topical ophthalmic drops: naphazoline HCl 0.1%.

Dose   1–2 drops four times per day, as needed for symptoms.

Contraindications   In patients with anatomically narrow angle or NAG or if hypersensitivity to the product or any of its components exists.

Warnings   Patients under therapy with MAOIs may experience a severe hypertensive crisis if given a sympathomimetic drug. Use in children, especially infants, may result in CNS depression leading to coma and marked reduction in body temperature. Concurrent use of maprotiline or TCAs and naphazoline may potentiate the pressor effect of naphazoline.

Adverse Reactions   *Ocular*: mydriasis, increased redness, irritation, discomfort, blurring, punctate keratitis, lacrimation, increased IOP. *Systemic*: dizziness, headache, nausea, sweating, nervousness, drowsiness, weakness, hypertension, cardiac irregularities, hyperglycemia.

Pregnancy Category   C.

Drug Interactions   It is not known whether this drug is excreted in human milk. Safety and effectiveness in pediatric patients have not been established.

Natamycin

Brand Name   Natacyn.

Class of Drug   Antifungal. Interferes with fungal cell membrane.

Indications   Fungal blepharitis, conjunctivitis, keratitis caused by susceptible organisms (yeast and filamentous fungi, including *Candida, Aspergillus, Cephalosporium, Fusarium, Penicillium*).

Dosage Form   Topical ophthalmic drops: natamycin ophthalmic suspension 5%.

Dose   1 drop hourly or 2-h for the first 3–4 days; may be reduced to six to eight times per day; generally continued for 14–21 days..

Contraindications   In patients hypersensitive to the product or any of its components.

Warnings   There have only been a limited number of cases in which natamycin has been used; therefore, it is possible that adverse reactions of which we have no knowledge at present may occur. Patients should be monitored at least two times per weekly. Should suspicion of drug toxicity occur, the drug should be discontinued.

Adverse Reactions	Conjunctival chemosis, hyperemia.
Pregnancy Category	C.
Drug Interactions	It is not known whether this drug is excreted in human milk. Safety and effectiveness in pediatric patients have not been established.

Nedocromil Sodium

Brand Name	Alocril.
Class of Drug	Mast cell stabilizer.
Indications	Itching associated with allergic conjunctivitis.
Dosage Form	Topical ophthalmic drops: nedocromil sodium ophthalmic solution 2%.
Dose	1 or 2 drops two times per day throughout the period of exposure.
Contraindications	In patients hypersensitive to the product or any of its components.
Adverse Reactions	Headache, ocular burning, irritation and stinging, unpleasant taste, nasal congestion, asthma, conjunctivitis, eye redness, photophobia, rhinitis.
Pregnancy Category	B.
Drug Interactions	It is not known whether this drug is excreted in human milk. Safety and effectiveness in children younger than 3 years of age have not been established.

Neomycin Sulfate

Brand Name	Cortisporin; NeoDecadron Neosporin; Poly-Pred; Dexacine; Neomycin and Polymyxin B Sulfates and Bacitracin Zinc; Neomycin and Polymyxin B Sulfates; Bacitracin Zinc and Hydrocortisone; Neomycin and Polymyxin B Sulfates and Dexamethasone; Neomycin and Polymyxin B Sulfates and Gramicidin.
Class of Drug	Antibiotic. Inhibits protein synthesis by binding to ribosomal RNA.
Indications	Superficial infections, such as conjunctivitis, keratitis, blepharitis. *S. aureus, E. coli, H. influenzae, Klebsiella/Enterobacter*

spp., *Neisseria* spp., *P. aeruginosa*. Does not provide adequate coverage against *S. marcescens* and streptococci, including *S. pneumoniae*.

Dosage Form
Topical ophthalmic ointment: each gram contains neomycin sulfate equivalent to 3.5 mg neomycin base. *Topical ophthalmic solution or suspension*: contain 0.35% neomycin base.

Dose
1 or 2 drops every 3 or 4 h, depending on the severity of the condition. Suspension may be used more frequently if necessary.

Contraindications
In patients who have shown hypersensitivity to the product or any of its components. Hypersensitivity to the antibiotic component occurs at a higher rate than for other components.

Warnings
Not for injection into the eye. Allergic cross-reactions may occur, which could prevent use of any or all of the following antibiotics for the treatment of future infections: kanamycin, paromomycin, streptomycin, and possibly gentamicin.

Adverse Reactions
Cutaneous sensitization; itching, reddening, and edema of the conjunctiva and eyelid. More serious hypersensitivity reactions, including anaphylaxis, have been reported rarely.

Pregnancy Category
C.

Drug Interactions
It is not known whether this drug is excreted in human milk. Safety and effectiveness in pediatric patients have not been established.

Ofloxacin

Brand Name	Ocuflox.
Class of Drug	Antibiotic. Bactericidal effect on susceptible bacterial cells by inhibiting DNA gyrase.
Indications	Bacterial conjunctivitis, bacterial corneal ulcer. Aerobes, gram-positive—*S. aureus, S. epidermidis, S. pneumoniae*. Aerobes, gram-negative—*E. cloacae, H. influenzae, P. mirabilis, P. aeruginosa, S. marcescens*. Anaerobic species—*Propionibacterium acnes*.
Dosage Form	Topical ophthalmic drops: ofloxacin ophthalmic solution 0.3%.
Dose	*Bacterial conjunctivitis*: 1–2 drops every 2–4 h. *Bacterial corneal ulcer*: 1–2 drops every 30 min while awake. Awaken at approximately 4 and 6 h after retiring and instill 1–2 drops.
Contraindications	In patients hypersensitive to the product or any of its components.
Warnings	Not for injection. Serious and occasionally fatal hypersensitivity (anaphylactic) reactions, some following the first dose, have been reported in patients receiving systemic quinolones, including ofloxacin. Some reactions were accompanied by cardiovascular collapse, loss of consciousness, angioedema (including laryngeal, pharyngeal, or facial edema), airway obstruction, dyspnea, urticaria, and itching. A rare occurrence of Stevens–Johnson syndrome, which progressed to toxic epidermal necrolysis, was reported in a patient who was receiving topical ophthalmic ofloxacin. If an allergic reaction occurs, discontinue the drug. Serious acute hypersensitivity reactions may require immediate emergency treatment. Oxygen and airway management, including intubation, should be administered as clinically indicated.
Adverse Reactions	Transient ocular burning or discomfort, stinging, redness, itching, chemical conjunctivitis/keratitis, ocular/periocular/facial edema, foreign-body sensation, photophobia, blurred vision, tearing, dryness, eye pain. Rare reports of dizziness and nausea have been received.
Pregnancy Category	C.
Drug Interactions	It is not known whether this drug is excreted in human milk following topical ophthalmic administration. Because of the potential for serious adverse reactions in nursing infants, a decision should be made whether to discontinue nursing or to discontinue the drug, taking into account the importance of the drug to the mother. Safety and effectiveness in infants younger than 1 year of age have not been established.

Olopatadine Hydrochloride

Brand Name	Patanol.
Class of Drug	Selective H_1-receptor antagonist and inhibitor of histamine release.
Indications	Allergic conjunctivitis.
Dosage Form	Topical ophthalmic drops: olopatadine hydrochloride ophthalmic solution 0.1%.
Dose	1 drop two times per day at an interval of 6–8 h.
Contraindications	In patients hypersensitive to the product or any of its components.
Warnings	For topical use only; not for injection or oral use.
Adverse Reactions	Headaches, asthenia, blurred vision, burning or stinging, cold syndrome, dry eye, foreign-body sensation, hyperemia, hypersensitivity, keratitis, lid edema, nausea, pharyngitis, pruritus, rhinitis, sinusitis, taste perversion.
Pregnancy Category	C.
Drug Interactions	It is not known whether topical ocular administration could result in sufficient systemic absorption to produce detectable quantities in the human milk. Safety and effectiveness in pediatric patients younger than 3 years of age have not been established.

Oxymetazoline Hydrochloride

Brand Name	Visine L.R.
Class of Drug	Vasoconstrictor.
Indications	Redness of the eye due to minor eye irritations.
Dosage Form	Topical ophthalmic drops: oxymetazoline HCl 0.025%.
Dose	1 or 2 drops; may be repeated as needed every 6 h.
Contraindications	In patients hypersensitive to the product or any of its components or if patient has NAG.
Adverse Reactions	Changes in vision, eye pain, redness.
Pregnancy Category	C.
Drug Interactions	It is not known whether this drug is excreted in human milk. Safety and effectiveness in pediatric patients have not been established.

Peg-200 Glyceryl Tallowate

Brand Name   Eye Scrub.
Class of Drug   Extra-gentle, nonirritating, hypoallergenic sterile eyelid cleanser.
Indications   Itching due to chronic blepharitis.
Dosage Form   Topical ophthalmic solution.
Dose   1. Apply a warm compress to closed eyes for several minutes before cleansing. 2. Wet, but do not saturate, a cleansing pad with cleanser and rub to work up a lather. 3. Rub the pad several times along the upper and lower lid at the base where the lashes grow out. Be careful not to rub the surface of the eye. Close the eye and rub the pad vigorously across the eyelashes several times. 4. Thoroughly rinse both eyes with warm water and pat dry.
Contraindications   In patients with known allergies to the product or any of its components.
Adverse Reactions   Excessive dryness, itching, redness, swelling, irritation.

Peg-200 Hydrogenated Glyceryl Palmate

Brand Name   Eye Scrub.
Class of Drug   See »Peg-200 Glyceryl Tallowate.«.
Indications   See »Peg-200 Glyceryl Tallowate.«
Dosage Form   Premoistened pads.
Dose   See »Peg-200 Glyceryl Tallowate.«
Contraindications   See »Peg-200 Glyceryl Tallowate.«
Adverse Reactions   See »Peg-200 Glyceryl Tallowate.«

Pegaptanib

Brand Name   Macugen.
Class of Drug   Selective vascular endothelial growth factor (VEGF) inhibitor.
Indications   Neovascular (wet) age-related macular degeneration (AMD).
Dosage Form   Injection 0.3 mg.
Dose   IV 0.3 mg once every 6 weeks.
Contraindications   In patients with ocular or periocular infections.
Warnings   Intravitreous injections have been associated with endophthalmitis. Proper aseptic injection technique should always be utilized. In addition, patient should be monitored during

the week following injection to permit early treatment should an infection occur.

Adverse Reactions *Ocular*: anterior chamber inflammation, blurred vision, cataract, conjunctival hemorrhage, corneal edema, eye discharge, eye irritation, eye pain, hypertension, increased IOP, ocular discomfort, punctuate keratitis, reduced visual acuity, visual disturbance, vitreous floaters (10–40% of patients). Blepharitis, conjunctivitis, photopsia, vitreous disorder (6–10% of patients). Allergic conjunctivitis, conjunctival edema, corneal abrasion, corneal deposits, corneal epithelium disorder, endophthalmitis, eye inflammation, eye swelling, eyelid irritation, meibomitis, mydriasis, periorbital hematoma, retinal edema, vitreous hemorrhage (1–5%) of patients. *Nonocular*: bronchitis, diarrhea, dizziness, headache, nausea, UTI (6–10% of patients). Arthritis, bone spur, carotid artery occlusion, stroke, chest pain, contact dermatitis, contusion, diabetes mellitus, dyspepsia, hearing loss, pleural effusion, transient ischemic attack, urinary retention, vertigo, vomiting (1–5% of patients).

Pregnancy Category B.

Pemirolast Potassium

Brand Name   Alamast.
Class of Drug   Mast cell stabilizer.
Indications   Prevention of itching due to allergic conjunctivitis.
Dosage Form   Topical ophthalmic drops: pemirolast potassium ophthalmic solution 0.1%.
Dose   1–2 drops four times per day.
Contraindications   In patients hypersensitive to the product or any of its components.
Warnings   For topical ophthalmic use only.Not for injection or oral use.
Adverse Reactions   *Ocular*: dry eye, foreign-body sensation, ocular discomfort. *Nonocular*: back pain, bronchitis, cough, dysmenorrhea, fever.
Pregnancy Category C.
Drug Interactions   It is not known whether this drug is excreted in human milk. Caution should be exercised administered to a nursing woman. Safety and effectiveness in pediatric patients younger than 3 years of age have not been established.

Penicillin G

Brand Name	Bicillin; Pfizerpen.
Class of Drug	Antibiotic.
Indications	Bejel, chorea prevention, glomerulonephritis, latent early syphilis, latent late bejel, latent late syphilis, latent late yaws, neurosyphilis, pharyngitis due to S. pyogenes, pinta, primary genital syphilis, rheumatic fever prevention, secondary syphilis, streptococcal tonsillitis, symptomatic congenital syphilis, syphilis, tertiary bejel, tertiary syphilis, tertiary yaws, yaws. *Note*: Severe pneumonia, empyema, bacteremia, pericarditis, meningitis, and peritonitis are better treated with penicillin G sodium or potassium during the acute stage.
Dosage Form	See section on Injectable Antibiotics.
Dose	Ranging from four doses of 0.6–1.2 MIU to six doses of 4 MIU i.v.
Contraindications	In patients with a previous hypersensitivity reaction to any penicillin. Significant—C. difficile colitis, infectious mononucleosis, renal disease.
Warnings	Serious and occasionally fatal hypersensitivity (anaphylactic) reactions have been reported in patients on penicillin therapy. These reactions are more likely to occur in individuals with a history of penicillin hypersensitivity and/or a history of sensitivity to multiple allergens. There have been reports of individuals with a history of penicillin hypersensitivity who have experienced severe reactions when treated with cephalosporins. Before initiating therapy with Bicillin C-R, careful inquiry should be made concerning previous hypersensitivity reactions to penicillins, cephalosporins, and other allergens. If an allergic reaction occurs, Bicillin C-R should be discontinued and appropriate therapy instituted. Serious anaphylactic reactions require immediate emergency treatment with epinephrine, oxygen, intravenous steroids. Airway management, including intubation, should also be administered as indicated. Care should be taken to avoid i.v. or intra-arterial administration or injection into or near major peripheral nerves or blood vessels since such injections may produce neurovascular damage.
Adverse Reactions	*Most frequent*: diarrhea, headache, nausea, oral candidiasis, vomiting, vulvovaginal candidiasis. *Less frequent*: allergic reactions, anaphylaxis, dyspnea, exfoliative dermatitis, facial edema, hypotension, pruritus, serum sickness, skin rash, urticaria. *Rare*: drug toxin-related hepatitis, interstitial nephritis, leukopenia, mental changes, neutropenia, seizure disorder, thrombocytopenia, C. difficile colitis.
Pregnancy Category	B.

Drug Interactions   Soluble penicillin G is excreted in human milk. <u>May cause sensitization, diarrhea, or rash in nursing infant.</u> *Pediatric warning*: <u>undeveloped renal function will slow rate of elimination.</u>

Petrolatum, White

Brand Name   Refresh P.M.
Class of Drug   Basic ointment and protectant.
Indications   Strong temporary relief of burning, irritation, and discomfort due to the dryness of the eye.
Dosage Form   Ointment.
Dose   Apply a small amount (¼ in.) of ointment to the inside of the eyelid of affected eye(s).
Contraindications   In patients hypersensitive to the product or any of its components.
Warnings   For external use only. To avoid contamination, do not touch tip of container to any surface. Replace cap after use.
Adverse Reactions   N/A.
Drug Interactions   Not available.

Pheniramine Maleate

Brand Name   Naphcon-A; Visine-A.
Class of Drug   Antihistaminic.
Indications   Prevention of itching due to allergic conjunctivitis.
Dosage Form   Topical ophthalmic drops.
Dose   1 drop up to five times per day.
Contraindications   *Most significant*: acute asthma, lactating mother, newborn. *Significant*: benign prostatic hypertrophy, bladder neck obstruction, glaucoma, stenosing peptic ulcer, urinary retention. *Possibly significant*: disease of cardiovascular system, hypertension, hyperthyroidism.
Warnings   *Geriatric precaution*: <u>hypotension, hyperexcitability, anticholinergic side effects likely.</u>
Adverse Reactions   *Most frequent*: drowsiness, thick bronchial secretions. *Rare*: abdominal pain with cramps, acute confusional state, anorexia, blood dyscrasias, blurred vision, dizziness, dry nose, dry throat, dysuria, excitative psychosis, hyperhidrosis, nervousness, nightmares, skin photosensitivity, skin rash, tachycardia, tinnitus, visual changes, xerostomia.

Drug Interactions	In pregnancy, only when necessary; in nursing woman.*Pediatric absolute contraindication*: <u>Possible CNS excitation, convulsions in newborns.</u>
Pregnancy Category	C.

Phenylephrine Hydrochloride

Brand Name	Murocoll 2; AK-Nefrin; AK-Dilate; Mydfrin; Neo-Synephrine.
Class of Drug	Sympathomimetic, decongestant.
Indications	Diagnostic aid, mydriatic, relieve redness due to minor irritations.
Dosage Form	Topical ophthalmic solution: ophthalmic phenylephrine 0.12%, 2.5%, 10%.
Dose	*Eye examination*: Adults and children—1 drop 2.5%. *Before eye surgery*—Adults and teenagers: 1 drop 2.5% or 10%. Children—1 drop 2.5%. *Eye redness*: Adults and children—1 drop 0.12% every 3 or 4 h as needed.
Contraindications	The 2.5% and 10% strengths may worsen diabetes mellitus, heart or blood vessel disease, or high blood pressure.
Warnings	Children may be especially sensitive. The 10% strength is not recommended for use in infants. Also, the 2.5 and 10% strengths are not recommended for use in low-birth-weight infants.
Adverse Reactions	*Ocular*: burning or stinging, sensitivity to light watering. *Nonocular*: headache or brow ache; dizziness; fast, irregular, or pounding heartbeat; increased sweating; increase in blood pressure; paleness; trembling.
Drug Interactions	Studies of effects in pregnancy have not been done. It is not known whether this drug passes into human milk.
Pregnancy Category	C.

Pilocarpine Hydrochloride

Brand Name	Pilocar; Isopto Carpine; Pilocar-HS; Piloptic.
Class of Drug	Parasympathomimetic.
Indications	Antiglaucoma agent, miotic.
Dosage Form	Ocular system (eye insert). Ophthalmic gel. Topical ophthalmic drops.
Dose	*Insert*: Glaucoma—Adults and children, 1 ocular system every 7 days. *Gel*: Glaucoma—Adults and teenagers, once per day

at bedtime. *Drops*: Chronic glaucoma—Adults and children, 1 drop one to four times per day. Acute ACG—Adults and children, 1 drop every 5–10 min for three to six doses then 1 drop every 1–3 h until eye pressure is reduced.

Contraindications   Asthma.

Warnings   Ocular formulations have been reported to cause visual blurring that may result in decreased visual acuity, especially at night and in patients with central lens changes, and to cause impairment of depth perception. Caution should be advised while driving at night or performing hazardous activities in reduced lighting

Adverse Reactions   Eye irritation, headache or brow ache, eye pain, blurred vision or change in near or far vision, decreased night vision, troubled breathing, wheezing, watering of mouth, increased sweating, muscle tremors, nausea, vomiting, diarrhea.

Pregnancy Category   C.

Drug Interactions   Studies on effects in pregnancy have not been done. It is not known whether this drug passes into human milk.

Piperacillin

Brand Name   Pipracil.

Class of Drug   Antibiotic.

Indications   Intra-abdominal infections—including hepatobiliary and surgical infections caused by *E coli*; *P aeruginosa*; enterococci; *Clostridium* spp; anaerobic cocci; *Bacteroides* spp, including *B. fragilis*. UTIs—caused by *E coli*; *Klebsiella* spp; *P. aeruginosa*; *Proteus* spp, including *P. mirabilis*, enterococci. Gynecologic infections—including endometritis; pelvic inflammatory disease; pelvic cellulitis caused by *Bacteroides* spp, including *B. fragilis*, anaerobic cocci; *N. gonorrhoeae*; enterococci (*Streptococcus faecalis*). Septicemia—including bacteremia caused by *E. coli*, *Klebsiella* spp, *Enterobacter* spp, *Serratia* spp, *P. mirabilis*, *S. pneumoniae*, enterococci, *P. aeruginosa*, *Bacteroides* spp, anaerobic cocci. Lower respiratory tract infections—caused by *E. coli*, *Klebsiella* spp, *Enterobacter* spp, *P. aeruginosa*, *Serratia* spp, *H. influenzae*, *Bacteroides* spp, anaerobic cocci; although improvement has been noted in patients with cystic fibrosis, lasting bacterial eradication may not necessarily be achieved. Skin and skin structure infections—caused by *E. coli*; *Klebsiella* spp; *Serratia* spp; *Acinetobacter* spp; *Enterobacter* spp; *P. aeruginosa*; indole-positive *Proteus* spp; *P. mirabilis*; *Bacteroides* spp, including *B. fragilis*, anaerobic cocci, enterococci. Bone and joint infections—caused by *P. aeruginosa*, enterococci,

	Bacteroides spp, anaerobic cocci. Gonococcal infections—has been effective in the treatment of uncomplicated gonococcal urethritis.

Dosage Form See section on Antibiotics.

Dose May be administered i.m. or i.v. or given in a 3- to 5-min i.v. injection. Usual dosage for serious infections is 3–4 g given every 4–6 h as a 20- to 30-min. infusion. For serious infections, the i.v. route should be used. Should not be mixed with an aminoglycoside in a syringe or infusion bottle since this can result in inactivation of the aminoglycoside. Maximum daily dose for adults is usually 24 g although higher doses have been used; i.m. injections should be limited to 2 g per injection site; this route of administration has been used primarily in the treatment of patients with uncomplicated gonorrhea and UTIs.

Contraindications In patients with a history of allergic reactions to any of the penicillins and/or cephalosporins.*Significant*: infectious mononucleosis, renal disease, *C. difficile* colitis. *Possibly significant*: hemorrhagic diathesis.

Warnings Serious and occasionally fatal hypersensitivity (anaphylactic) has been reported in patients receiving therapy with penicillins. These reactions are more apt to occur in persons with a history of sensitivity to multiple allergens. There have been reports of patients with a history of penicillin hypersensitivity who experienced severe hypersensitivity reactions when treated with a cephalosporin. Before initiating therapy, careful inquiry should be made concerning previous hypersensitivity reactions to penicillins, cephalosporins, and other allergens. If an allergic reaction occurs during therapy, the antibiotic should be discontinued. The usual agents (antihistamines, pressor amines, corticosteroids) should be readily available.Serious anaphylactoid reactions require immediate emergency treatment with epinephrine. Oxygen and i.v. corticosteroids and airway management, including intubation, should also be administered as necessary.

Adverse Reactions *Most frequent*: diarrhea, headache, nausea, oral candidiasis, vomiting, vulvovaginal candidiasis. *Less frequent*: allergic reactions, anaphylaxis, dyspnea, exfoliative dermatitis, facial edema, hypotension, pruritus, serum sickness, skin rash, urticaria. *Rare*: drug toxin-related hepatitis, interstitial nephritis, leukopenia, mental changes, neutropenia, seizure disorder, thrombocytopenia, *C. difficile* colitis.

Pregnancy Category B.

Drug Interactions Caution should be exercised when administered to nursing mothers. It is excreted in low concentrations in human milk. Poor oral absorption; possible sensitization, diarrhea or rash in infants. Dosages for children younger than 12 years of age have not been established. Safety in neonates is not known. *Warning*: Undeveloped renal function will slow rate of elimination.

Polyethylene Glycol

Brand Name   Systane; Advanced Relief Visine; Visine Tears; Visine Tears Preservative Free.

Class of Drug   Lubricant.

Indications   Relief of redness of the eye due to minor irritations; protection against further irritation.

Dosage Form   Topical ophthalmic drops: polyethylene glycol 400, 0.4–1%.

Dose   1 or 2 drops up to four times per day.

Contraindications   In patients hypersensitive to the product or any of its components.

Pregnancy Category C.

Polymyxin B Sulfate

Brand Name   Cortisporin; Neosporin; Poly-Pred; Polysporin; Polytrim; Bacitracin Zinc and Polymyxin B Sulfates; Dexacine; Neomycin and Polymyxin B Sulfates and Bacitracin Zinc; Neomycin and Polymyxin B Sulfates; Bacitracin Zinc and Hydrocortisone; Neomycin and Polymyxin B Sulfates and Dexamethasone; Neomycin and Polymyxin B Sulfates and Gramicidin; Polymyxin B Sulfate and Trimethoprim Sulfate; AK-Poly-Bac; Polycin-B.

Class of Drug   Antibiotic.

Indications   Bacterial conjunctivitis, bacterial corneal ulcer, *S. aureus*, *E. coli*, *H. influenzae*, *Klebsiella/Enterobacter* spp., *Neisseria* spp., *P. aeruginosa*. No adequate coverage against *S. marcescens*; streptococci, including *S. pneumoniae*.

Dosage Form   Topical ophthalmic drops and ointment.

Dose   *Eye*: 1 or 2 drops to affected eye(s) every 3–4 h, or more frequently as required. *Eye lids*: 1 or 2 drops to affected eye(s) every 3–4 h, close the eye, and rub the excess on the lids and lid margins.

Contraindications   In patients hypersensitive to the product or any of its components.

Warnings   Avoid wearing contact lenses when using these eye preparations. Application to large areas of skin will increase the risk of side effects, such as hearing damage. Prolonged use of an anti-infective may result in the development of superinfection due to microorganisms, including fungi, resistant to that anti-infective.

Adverse Reactions   Cutaneous sensitization.

Drug Interactions	C.
Drug Interactions	*Pregnancy*: possibly safe. *Lactation*: precaution—no data available.

Polysorbate 80

Brand Name	Refresh Endura.
Class of Drug	Lubricant.
Indications	Relief of burning, irritation, and discomfort due to dryness of the eye or exposure to wind or sun.
Dosage Form	Topical ophthalmic drops: polysorbate 80, 1%.
Dose	1–2 drops as needed.
Contraindications	In patients hypersensitive to the product or any of its components.
Warnings	For external use only. To avoid contamination, do not touch tip of container to any surface. Do not reuse. Once opened, discard. Do not touch unit dose tip to eye. Do not use if solution changes color.

Polyvinylpyrrolidone

Brand Name	See »Povidone.«

Povidone

Brand Name	Advanced Relief Visine.
Class of Drug	Lubricant.
Indications	Relief of redness of the eye due to minor irritations and dryness.
Dosage Form	Topical ophthalmic drops: povidone 1%.
Dose	1–2 drops up to four times per day.
Contraindications	In patients hypersensitive to the product or any of its components.
Warnings	Specifically applied to Advanced Relief Visine. Ask a doctor before use if you have NAG. When using this product, pu-

pils may become enlarged temporarily. Overuse may cause
more eye redness. Remove contact lenses before using. Do
not use if solution changes color or becomes cloudy. To avoid
contamination, do not touch tip of container to any surface.
Replace cap after each use. Stop use and ask a doctor if you
experience eye pain or changes in vision, if redness or irritation lasts, or condition worsens or lasts more than 72 h.

Pregnancy Category   C.

Povidone Iodine

Brand Name	Betadine 5%.
Class of Drug	Broad-spectrum microbicide.
Indications	Prepping of the periocular region (lids, brow, cheek) and irrigation of the ocular surface (cornea, conjunctiva, palpebral fornices).
Dosage Form	Topical ophthalmic drops: povidone-iodine 5% (0.5% available iodine).
Dose	1. Saturate sterile cotton-tipped applicator to prep lashes and lid margins using one or more applicators per lid; repeat once. 2. Saturate sterile prep sponge or other suitable material to prep lids, brow, and cheek in a circular, ever-expanding fashion until the entire field is covered; repeat prep three times. 3. While separating the lids, irrigate the cornea, conjunctiva, and palpebral fornices using a sterile bulb syringe. 4. After the solution has been left in contact for 2 min, sterile saline solution in a bulb syringe should be used to flush the residual from the cornea, conjunctiva, and palpebral fornices.
Contraindications	In patients hypersensitive to the product or any of its components.
Warnings	<u>Not for intraocular injection or irrigation</u>. No studies are available in patients with thyroid disorders; therefore, caution is advised in these patients due to the possibility of iodine absorption.
Adverse Reactions	Local sensitivity.
Pregnancy Category	C.
Drug Interactions	Because of the potential for serious adverse reactions in nursing infants, a decision should be made to discontinue nursing or discontinue the drug, taking into account the importance of the drug to the mother. Safety and effectiveness in pediatric patients have not been established.

Prednisolone Acetate

Brand Name   Blephamide; Poly-Pred; Pred Forte; Pred Mild; Pred-G; Meti-
                       myd; Econopred; Econopred Plus.
Class of Drug   Glucocorticoid; three to five times the anti-inflammatory po-
                       tency of hydrocortisone.
Indications   In inflammatory conditions of the palpebral and bulbar con-
                       junctiva, cornea, and anterior segment of the globe where
                       the inherent risk of corticosteroid use in certain infective con-
                       junctivitides is accepted to obtain a diminution in edema and
                       inflammation. In chronic anterior uveitis and corneal injury
                       from chemical, radiation, or thermal burns or penetration of
                       foreign bodies.
Dosage Form   Topical ophthalmic drops: prednisolone acetate 1%.
Dose   2 drops to the conjunctival sac every 4 h during the day and
                       at bedtime.
Contraindications Corticosteroids should be used with caution in the presence
                       of glaucoma. IOP should be checked frequently. Contraindi-
                       cated in most viral diseases of the cornea and conjunctiva,
                       dendritic keratitis, vaccinia, and varicella, and also in myco-
                       bacterial infection of the eye and fungal diseases of ocular
                       structures.
Warnings   Not for injection into the eye. Topical steroids are not effective
                       in mustard gas keratitis and Sjögren's keratoconjunctivitis.
Adverse Reactions Elevation of IOP with possible development of glaucoma and
                       infrequent optic nerve damage, posterior subcapsular cata-
                       ract formation, and delayed wound healing. May suppress
                       the host response and thus increase hazard of secondary
                       ocular infections. In diseases causing thinning of the cornea
                       or sclera, perforation has been known to occur with the use
                       of topical corticosteroids. In acute purulent conditions of the
                       eye, corticosteroids may mask infection or enhance existing
                       infection. Corticosteroid-containing preparations can also
                       cause acute anterior uveitis or perforation of the globe. My-
                       driasis, loss of accommodation, and ptosis have occasionally
                       been reported following local use of corticosteroids. Alt-
                       hough systemic effects are extremely uncommon, there have
                       been rare occurrences of systemic hypercorticoidism after
                       use of topical corticosteroids.
Pregnancy Category C.
Drug Interactions It is not known whether topical administration of corticoste-
                       roids could result in sufficient systemic absorption to produ-
                       ce detectable quantities in human milk. Safety and effective-
                       ness in pediatric patients younger than 6 years of age have
                       not been established.

Prednisolone Sodium Phosphate

Brand Name	Inflamase Forte 1%; Inflamase Mild 1/8%; Vasocidin; AK-Pred.
Class of Drug	Glucocorticoid, anti-inflammatory agent.
Indications	See »Prednisolone Acetate.«
Dosage Form	Topical ophthalmic drops 1/8–1%.
Dose	See »Prednisolone Acetate.«
Contraindications	See »Prednisolone Acetate.«
Warnings	See »Prednisolone Acetate.«
Adverse Reactions	See »Prednisolone Acetate.«
Pregnancy Category	See »Prednisolone Acetate.«
Drug Interactions	See »Prednisolone Acetate.«

Prilocaine

Brand Name	Citanest.
Class of Drug	Local anesthetic.
Indications	Local anesthesia.
Dosage Form	Parenteral for injection.
Dose	Maximum dose 5.7 mg/kg body weight. Rapid onset; lasts for 1.5–3 h.
Contraindications	Patients with a known history of hypersensitivity to local anesthetics of the amide type or to other components this product. Patients with congenital or idiopathic methemoglobinemia.
Warnings	Local anesthetics should only be employed by clinicians who are well versed in diagnosis and management of dose-related toxicity and other acute emergencies that might arise from the block to be employed and then only after ensuring the immediate availability of oxygen, other resuscitative drugs, cardiopulmonary equipment, and the personnel needed for proper management of toxic reactions and related emergencies. To minimize the likelihood of intravascular injection, aspiration should be performed before the local anesthetic solution is injected. If blood is aspirated, the needle must be repositioned until no return of blood can be elicited by aspiration. Citanest 4% Forte contains sodium metabisulfite, a sulfite that may cause allergic-type reactions, including anaphylactic symptoms and life-threatening or less-severe asthmatic episodes in certain susceptible people. Sulfite sensitivity is seen more frequently in asthmatic than in nonasthmatic people.

Adverse Reactions

CNS: Circumoral paresthesia, lightheadedness, nervousness, apprehension, euphoria, confusion, dizziness, drowsiness, hyperacusis, tinnitus, blurred vision, vomiting, sensations of heat, cold or numbness, twitching, tremors, convulsions, unconsciousness, and respiratory depression and arrest. Excitatory manifestations may be very brief or may not occur at all, in which case the first manifestation of toxicity may be drowsiness merging into unconsciousness and respiratory arrest. Drowsiness following the administration of prilocaine is usually an early sign of a high prilocaine plasma level and may occur as a consequence of rapid absorption. *Cardiovascular*: usually depressant and are characterized by bradycardia, hypotension, arrhythmia, and cardiovascular collapse, which may lead to cardiac arrest. *Allergic*: characterized by cutaneous lesions, urticaria, edema, or in the most severe instances, anaphylactic shock. *Neurologic*: persistent paresthesia and sensory disturbances. *Methemoglobinemia*: Cyanosis due to the formation of methemoglobin may occur after administration. Repeated administration, even in relatively small doses, can lead to clinically overt methemoglobinemia. Note: Even low concentrations of methemoglobin may interfere with pulse oximetry readings, indicating false low oxygen saturation.

Pregnancy Category

B.

Drug Interactions

Should be used with caution in patients receiving other agents structurally related to amide-type local anesthetics since the toxic effects are additive. Citanest 4% Forte, which contains epinephrine, should not be used concomitantly with ergot-type oxytocic drugs because a severe, persistent hypertension may occur and cerebrovascular and cardiac accidents are possible. Likewise, Citanest 4% Forte or solutions containing Citanest 4% Plain and another vasoconstrictor should be used with extreme caution in patients receiving MAOIs or antidepressants of the triptyline or imipramine types. Phenothiazines and butyrophenones may reduce or reverse the pressor effect of epinephrine. If sedatives are employed to reduce patient apprehension, they should be used in reduced doses. Solutions containing epinephrine should be used with caution in patients undergoing general anesthesia with inhalation agents such as halothane due to the risk of serious cardiac arrhythmias. Possibly safe in pregnancy. It is not known whether this drug or its metabolites are excreted in human milk. Safety and effectiveness in pediatric patients have not been established.

Procaine

Brand Name	Novocaine.
Class of Drug	Local anesthetic.
Indications	Local anesthesia.
Dosage Form	Parenteral for injection.
Dose	Maximum dose 7 mg/kg body weight. Slow onset; last for 30–45 min.
Contraindications	*Most significant*: infection at site. *Significant*: disease of cardiovascular system, myasthenia gravis, plasma cholinesterase deficiency. *Possibly significant*: liver disease, renal disease.
Warnings	Local anesthetics should only be employed by clinicians who are well versed in diagnosis and management of dose-related toxicity and other acute emergencies that might arise from the block to be employed and then only after ensuring the immediate availability of oxygen, other resuscitative drugs, cardiopulmonary equipment, and the personnel needed for proper management of toxic reactions and related emergencies. To minimize the likelihood of intravascular injection, aspiration should be performed before the local anesthetic solution is injected. If blood is aspirated, the needle must be repositioned until no return of blood can be elicited by aspiration.
Adverse Reactions	Allergic reactions, anaphylaxis, CNS toxicity, erythema, methemoglobinemia, myocardial dysfunction, nausea, pruritus, skin rash, sneezing, urticaria, vasodilation of blood vessels, vomiting.
Pregnancy Category	C.
Drug Interactions	Possibly safe in pregnancy. It is not known whether this drug or its metabolites are excreted in human milk. Safety and effectiveness in pediatric patients have not been established.

Proparacaine Hydrochloride

Brand Name	Ophthetic; Alcaine; Parcaine.
Class of Drug	Topical local anesthetic.
Indications	Corneal anesthesia of short duration, e.g., tonometry, gonioscopy, removal of corneal foreign bodies, short corneal and conjunctival procedures lasting approximately 10–20 min.
Dosage Form	Topical ophthalmic drops: proparacaine HCl 0.5%.
Dose	*Removal of foreign bodies and sutures and for tonometry*: 1–2 drops (in single instillations). *Short corneal and conjunctival procedures*: 1 drop every 5–10 min for five to seven doses.

Contraindications	In patients with a known hypersensitivity to the product or any of its components.
Warnings	Prolonged use of a topical ocular anesthetic is not recommended; may produce permanent corneal opacification with accompanying visual loss.
Adverse Reactions	Stinging, burning, and conjunctival redness. A rare, severe, immediate-type, apparently hyperallergic, corneal reaction characterized by acute, intense, and diffuse epithelial keratitis, a gray, ground-glass appearance, sloughing of large areas of necrotic epithelium, corneal filaments and, sometimes, iritis with descemetitis has been reported. Contact dermatitis with drying and fissuring of the fingertips.
Pregnancy Category	C.
Drug Interactions	It is not known whether this drug is excreted in human milk.

Propylene Glycol

Brand Name	Systane.
Class of Drug	Lubricant.
Indications	Temporary relief of burning and irritation due to dryness of the eye.
Dosage Form	Topical ophthalmic drops: propylene glycol 0.3%.
Dose	1–2 drops as needed.
Warnings	If you experience eye pain, changes in vision, continued redness, or irritation of the eye, or if the condition worsens or persists for more than 72 h, discontinue use and consult a doctor. Do not use if product changes color or becomes cloudy or if you are sensitive to any component of this product. To avoid contamination, do not touch tip of container to any surface. Replace cap after each use. Keep this and all drugs out of the reach of children. In case of accidental ingestion, seek professional assistance or contact a poison control center immediately

Rimexolone

Brand Name Vexol.

Class of Drug Corticosteroid.

Indications First choice in steroid responders. Inflammatory conditions of the palpebral and bulbar conjunctiva, cornea, and anterior segment of the globe where the inherent risk of corticosteroid use in certain infective conjunctivitides is accepted to obtain a diminution in edema and inflammation. Chronic anterior uveitis and corneal injury from chemical, radiation, or thermal burns or penetration of foreign bodies.

Dosage Form Topical ophthalmic drops: rimexolone.

Dose 1 or 2 drops four times per day or more often as needed.

Contraindications Corticosteroids should be used with caution in the presence of glaucoma; IOP should be checked frequently. In most viral diseases of the cornea and conjunctiva dendritic keratitis, vaccinia, and varicella; in mycobacterial infection of the eye and fungal diseases of ocular structures.

Warnings Not for injection. Use in the treatment of herpes simplex infection requires great caution and frequent slit-lamp examinations. Prolonged use may result in ocular hypertension/glaucoma, damage to the optic nerve, defects in visual acuity and visual fields, and posterior subcapsular cataract formation. Prolonged use may also result in secondary ocular infections due to suppression of host response. Acute purulent infections of the eye may be masked or exacerbated by the presence of corticosteroid medication. In those diseases causing thinning of the cornea or sclera, perforation has been known to occur with topical steroids. It is advisable that IOP be checked frequently.

Adverse Reactions Blurred vision or other change in vision; eye discharge, discomfort, dryness, or tearing; eye redness, irritation, or pain; foreign-body sensation; itching, stuffy, or runny nose; swelling of the lining of the eyelids, lightheadedness or faintness, headache, brow ache; change in taste.

Pregnancy Category C.

Drug Interactions It is not known whether topical administration of corticosteroids could result in sufficient systemic absorption to produce detectable quantities in human milk. Safety and effectiveness in pediatric patients younger than six years of age have not been established.

Scopolamine Hydrochloride; Scopolamine Hydrobromide

Brand Name	Murocoll 2; Isopto Hyoscine.
Class of Drug	Cycloplegic, mydriatic.
Indications	Dilate pupil before eye examinations; before and after eye surgery; treat certain eye conditions, such as uveitis or posterior synechiae.
Dosage Form	Topical ophthalmic drops.
Dose	*Uveitis*: Adults and children—1 drop up to four times per day. *Eye examinations*: Adults—1 drop 1 h before the examination. Children—1 drop two times per day for 2 days before the examination. *Posterior synechiae*: Adults—1 drop every 10 min for three doses. *Before and after surgery*: Adults and children—1 drop one to four times per day.
Contraindications	In infants and young children and children with blond hair or blue eyes may be especially sensitive to the effects of atropine, homatropine, or scopolamine. This may increase the chance of side effects during treatment. Children should be given a lower strength of this medicine.
Warnings	Overdose is very dangerous for infants and children. May worsen brain damage (in children), Down syndrome (in children and adults), glaucoma or spastic paralysis (in children).
Adverse Reactions	*Ocular*: blurred vision, brief burning or stinging of the eyes, eye irritation not present before use of this medicine, increased sensitivity of eyes to light, swelling of the eyelids. *Nonocular*: clumsiness or unsteadiness; confusion or unusual behavior; dryness of skin; fast or irregular heartbeat; fever; flushing or redness of face; seeing, hearing, or feeling things that are not there; skin rash; slurred speech; swollen stomach in infants; thirst or unusual dryness of mouth; unusual drowsiness, tiredness, or weakness.
Pregnancy Category	C.
Drug Interactions	Studies on effects in pregnancy have not been done. It is not known whether this drug passes into human milk. Safety and effectiveness in pediatric patients have not been established.

Sirolimus

Brand Name	Rapamune.
Class of Drug	Inhibits T-lymphocyte activation and proliferation that occurs in response to antigenics and cytokines. Binds to the immunophilin FK-binding protein-12 (FKBP-12) to generate

an immunosuppressive complex. This complex binds to and inhibits activation of the mammalian target of rapamycin (mTOR), a key regulatory kinase. This inhibition suppresses cytokine-driven T-cell proliferation, inhibiting the progression from the G_1 to the S phase of the cell cycle.

Indications
Prophylaxis of organ rejection in patients receiving renal transplants. Shown to be effective treatment for autoimmune disease in experimental animals. No clinical trials in uveitis as yet. High potential, particularly in combination with CSA or other immunosuppressive agents, in the treatment of autoimmune uveitis.

Dosage Form
Oral solution: concentration of 1 mg/ml. *Tablets*: 1 mg, 2 mg.

Dose
A daily maintenance dose of 2 mg is recommended for use in renal transplant patients, with a loading dose of 6 mg; 2 mg of oral solution has been demonstrated to be clinically equivalent to 2 mg oral tablets and hence are interchangeable on a milligram-to-milligram basis. However, it is not known if higher doses of oral solution are clinically equivalent to higher doses of tablets on a milligram-to-milligram basis. Initial dosage in patients 13 years of age and older who weigh less than 40 kg should be adjusted, based on body surface area, to 1 mg/m^2 per day. Loading dose should be 3 mg/m^2. Recommended that maintenance dose be reduced by approximately one third in patients with hepatic impairment; not necessary to modify the loading dose. Dosage need not be adjusted because of impaired renal function.

Contraindications
In patients with hypersensitivity to the product or any of its components or any of its derivatives.

Warnings
Increased susceptibility to infection and possible development of lymphoma and other malignancies, particularly of the skin, may result from immunosuppression.

Adverse Reactions
Hyperlipidemia, hypercholesterolemia, anemia, thrombocytopenia, leucopenia, hypertension, rash, acne, arthralgia, diarrhea, constipation, hypokalemia, hypokalemia, hypophosphatemia, fever, headache, asthenia, back pain, chest pain, nausea and vomiting, dyspepsia, creatinine increase, edema, weight gain, insomnia, tremor, pharyngitis, dyspnea, UTI; elevation of triglycerides and cholesterol and decreases in platelets and hemoglobin occurred in a dose-related manner. Monitor serum lipid, CBC, and differential.

Pregnancy Category
C.

Drug Interactions
Safety and efficacy in pediatric patients younger than 13 years of age have not been established. Because of the effect of CSA, it is recommended that sirolimus be taken 4 h after administration of CSA oral solution and/or capsules. *Drugs that modify bioavailability*: ketoconazole, rifampin, diltiazem. *Drugs that may increase blood concentrations include*: Calcium channel blockers—nicardipine, verapamil. Antifungal agents—clotrimazole, fluconazole, itraconazole. Macrolide antibiotics—clarithromycin, erythromycin, troleandomycin.

Gastrointestinal prokinetic agents—cisapride, metoclopramide. Others—bromocriptine, cimetidine, danazol, HIV-protease inhibitors (e.g., ritonavir, indinavir). *Drugs that may decrease blood concentrations include*: Anticonvulsants—carbamazepine, phenobarbital, phenytoin. Antibiotics—rifabutin, rifapentine, St. John's wort. (This list is not all-inclusive.)

Sodium Chloride

Brand Name	Muro 128.
Class of Drug	Hyperosmotic.
Indications	Temporary relief of corneal edema.
Dosage Form	Topical ophthalmic drops: sodium chloride hypertonicity. Ophthalmic solution 2–5%.
Dose	1 or 2 drops every 3 or 4 h or as needed.
Warnings	Do not use except under the advice and supervision of a doctor. If you experience eye pain, changes in vision, continued redness or irritation, or if the condition worsens or persists, consult a doctor. To avoid contamination of the product, do not touch the tip of the container to any surface. Replace cap after using. May cause temporary burning and irritation. If the solution changes color or becomes cloudy, do not use. In case of accidental ingestion, seek professional assistance or contact a poison control center immediately.
Adverse Reactions	Temporary burning and irritation.

Sodium Hyaluronate

Brand Name	Amvisc Plus; Amvisc; Healon; Healon 5; Healon GV.
Class of Drug	Viscoelastic.
Indications	Surgical aid in ophthalmic anterior and posterior segment procedures, including extraction of cataract, implantation of an IOL, corneal transplantation surgery, glaucoma filtering surgery, surgical procedures to reattach the retina.
Dosage Form	High-molecular -eight polysaccharide for intraocular use 16 mg/ml sodium hyaluronate.
Dose	Intraocular use as needed.
Warnings	Should be removed from anterior chamber at the end of surgery.
Adverse Reactions	Increased IOP following surgery.

Sulfacetamide Sodium

Brand Name   Bleph-10; AK-Sulf; Blephamide; FML-S; Sulf-10; Vasocidin; Me-
                        timyd.
Class of Drug   Antibiotic.
Indications   Topical treatment of superficial infections of the external eye,
                        and adnexa, such as conjunctivitis, keratitis blepharitis.
Dosage Form   Topical ophthalmic drops. Topical ophthalmic ointment.
Dose   *Drops*: 1 drop every 1–3 h during the day and less often du-
                        ring the night. *Ointment*: four times per day and at bedtime.
Contraindications   Not be used with silver ophthalmic preparations since a che-
                        mical reaction may occur.
Adverse Reactions   Itching, redness, swelling, or other sign of irritation not pre-
                        sent before use of this medicine.
Pregnancy Category C.
Drug Interactions   Ophthalmic preparations have not been shown to cause pro-
                        blems in humans nor reported to cause problems in nursing
                        babies. Studies have been done only in adult patients, and
                        there is no specific information comparing use in children
                        with use in other age groups.

S

Tetracaine

Brand Name	Pontocaine.
Class of Drug	Local anesthetic.
Indications	Local anesthesia.
Dosage Form	Topical ophthalmic drops. Parenteral for injection.
Dose	Slow onset; lasts for 2–3 h.
Contraindications	Ocular infection; ocular inflammation. *Most significant*: infection at site. *Significant*: disease of cardiovascular system, myasthenia gravis, plasma cholinesterase deficiency. *Possibly significant*: liver disease, renal disease.
Warnings	High toxicity.
Adverse Reactions	*Ocular*: irritation, pain, redness, itching, allergic conjunctivitis, allergic reactions. *Nonocular*: cardiac arrhythmias, CNS depression, CNS toxicity, excitative psychosis, eyelid dermatitis, fatigue, hyperhidrosis, , pallor, allergic reactions, anaphylaxis, erythema, methemoglobinemia, myocardial dysfunction, nausea, pruritus, skin rash, sneezing, urticaria, vasodilation of blood vessels, vomiting.
Pregnancy Category	C.
Drug Interactions	Only when necessary in pregnancy. It is not known whether this drug or its metabolites are excreted in human milk. Relative contraindication: Risk of systemic toxicity possible in pediatric patients.

Tetracaine Hydrochloride

Brand Name	AK-T-Caine; Pontocaine.
Class of Drug	Local anesthetic.
Indications	Before certain procedures, such as measuring eye pressure, removing foreign objects or sutures, and performing certain examinations.
Dosage Form	Topical ophthalmic drops. Topical ophthalmic ointment.
Dose	1 drop or small amount of the ointment the lower eyelid.
Warnings	To be administered only by or under the immediate supervision of a doctor. After a local anesthetic is applied to the eye, do not rub or wipe the eye until the anesthetic has worn off and feeling returns; to do so may cause injury or damage to the eye. The effects of these medicines usually last long enough to treat injury or damage.
Adverse Reactions	Itching, pain, redness, or swelling of the eye or eyelid; watering; increased sweating; irregular heartbeat; muscle twitching or trembling; nausea or vomiting; shortness of breath or troubled breathing; unusual excitement, nervousness, or restlessness; unusual tiredness or weakness.

Pregnancy Category C.
Drug Interactions Although studies on effects in pregnancy have not been done in either humans or animals, this drug has not been reported to cause problems in humans. It is not known whether it passes into human milk. Although there is no specific information comparing use of ophthalmic anesthetics in children with use in other age groups, these medicines are not expected to cause different side effects or problems in children than they do in adults.

Tetrahydrozoline Hydrochloride

Brand Name Visine Original; Visine A.C.; Advanced Relief Visine; EyeSine; Murine Tears Plus.
Class of Drug Vasoconstrictor.
Indications Temporary relief of minor symptoms of ocular pruritus and conjunctival congestion.
Dosage Form Topical ophthalmic drops: tetrahydrozoline HCl 0.05%.
Dose 1 or 2 drops up to four times per day.
Warnings Ask a doctor before use if you have NAG. Pupils may become enlarged temporarily. Overuse may cause more eye redness. Remove contact lenses before using. Do not use if solution changes color or becomes cloudy. To avoid contamination, do not touch tip of container to any surface. Replace cap after each use. Stop use and ask a doctor if you experience eye pain, changes in vision occur, if redness or irritation of the eye lasts, or condition worsens or lasts more than 72 h.
Contraindications In patients with anatomically narrow angle or NAG or if hypersensitivity to the product or any of its components exists.
Adverse Reactions Mydriasis; increased redness, irritation, discomfort, blurring; punctate keratitis; lacrimation; increased IOP.
Pregnancy Category C.
Drug Interactions It is not known whether this drug is excreted in human milk. Safety and effectiveness in pediatric patients have not been established.

T

Ticarcillin disodium

Brand Name   Ticar.
Class of Drug   Antibiotic.
Indications   Septicemia—including bacteremia caused by beta-lacta-mase-producing strains of *Klebsiella* spp.*, *E. coli**, *S. aureus**, *P. aeruginosa** (or other *Pseudomonas* spp.*). LRIs—caused by beta-lactamase-producing strains of *S. aureus*, *H. influen-zae**, *Klebsiella* spp.*. Bone and joint infections—caused by beta-lactamase-producing strains of *S. aureus*. Skin and skin structure infections—caused by beta-lactamase-producing strains of *S. aureus*, *Klebsiella* spp.*, *E. coli**. UTIs (complicated and uncomplicated)—caused by beta-lactamase-producing strains of *E. coli*, *Klebsiella* spp., *P. aeruginosa** (or other *Pseu-domonas* spp.*), *Citrobacter* spp.*, *E. cloacae**, *S. marcescens**, *S. aureus*.* Gynecologic infections—endometritis caused by beta-lactamase-producing strains of *Bacteroides melanino-genicus**, *Enterobacter* spp. (including *E. cloacae**), *E. coli*, *K. pneumoniae**, *S. aureus*, or *S. epidermidis*. Intra-abdominal infections—peritonitis caused by beta-lactamase-producing strains of *E. coli*, *K. pneumoniae*, *B. fragilis**.

Dosage Form
Dose   Adult minimum:maximum: 4.0 g:24.0g.
Contraindications   In patients with a history of hypersensitivity reactions to any of the penicillins. *Significant*: infectious mononucleosis, renal disease, *C. difficile* colitis.
Warnings   Serious and occasionally fatal hypersensitivity (anaphylactic) reactions have been reported in patients on penicillin the-rapy. These reactions are more likely to occur in individuals with a history of penicillin hypersensitivity and/or a history of sensitivity to multiple allergens. There have been reports of individuals with a history of penicillin hypersensitivity who have experienced severe reactions when treated with cephalosporins. Before initiating therapy, careful inquiry should be made concerning previous hypersensitivity re-actions to penicillins, cephalosporins, or other allergens. If an allergic reaction occurs, therapy should be discontinued and the appropriate therapy instituted. Serious anaphylactic reactions require immediate emergency treatment with epinephrine. Oxygen, intravenous steroids, and airway ma-nagement, including intubation, should also be provided as indicated.
Adverse Reactions   *Most frequent*: diarrhea, headache, nausea, oral candidiasis, vomiting, vulvovaginal candidiasis. *Less frequent*: allergic re-actions, anaphylaxis, dyspnea, exfoliative dermatitis, facial edema, hypotension, pruritus, serum sickness, skin rash, ur-ticaria. *Rare*: drug toxin-related hepatitis, *C. difficile* colitis, in-

terstitial nephritis, leukopenia, mental changes, neutropenia, seizure disorder, thrombocytopenia.

Pregnancy Category B.

Drug Interactions It is not known whether this drug is excreted in human milk. <u>May cause sensitization, diarrhea, or rash in nursing infants.</u> Safety and effectiveness have been established in the age group of 3 months to 16 years. Use in these age groups is supported by evidence from adequate and well-controlled studies in adults, with additional efficacy, safety, and pharmacokinetic data from both comparative and noncomparative studies in pediatric patients. There are insufficient data to support use in pediatric patients younger than 3 months of age or for the treatment of septicemia and/or infections in the pediatric population where the suspected or proven pathogen is *H. influenzae* type B. *Warning*: <u>undeveloped renal function will slow rate of elimination.</u>

Timolol Hemihydrate, Timolol Maleate

Brand Name Betimol; Cosopt; Timolol GFS; Timoptic; Timoptic-XE.

Class of Drug Nonselective beta-blocking agent.

Indications In the treatment of elevated IOP in patients with ocular hypertension or OAG.

Dosage Form Topical ophthalmic drops: timolol 0.25%, 0.5%.

Dose 1 drop two times per day.

Contraindications See »Warnings.«

Warnings Severe respiratory and cardiac reactions, including death due to bronchospasm, in patients with asthma and, rarely, death in association with cardiac failure, have been reported following systemic or topical administration of beta-adrenergic-blocking agents. Should be administered with caution in patients subject to spontaneous hypoglycemia or diabetic patients. Beta-adrenergic-blocking agents may mask signs and symptoms of acute hypoglycemia and certain clinical signs (e.g., tachycardia) of hyperthyroidism. Patients suspected of developing thyrotoxicosis should be managed carefully to avoid abrupt withdrawal of beta-adrenergic-blocking agents, which might precipitate a thyroid storm.

Adverse Reactions *Ocular*: blepharitis, conjunctivitis, crusting, discomfort, foreign-body sensation, hyperemia, pruritus, tearing. *Cardiovascular*: bradycardia, arrhythmia, hypotension, hypertension, syncope, heart block, cerebral vascular accident, cerebral ischemia, cardiac failure, worsening of angina pectoris, palpitation, cardiac arrest, pulmonary edema, dizziness, edema, claudication, Raynaud's phenomenon, cold hands and feet.

Respiratory: bronchospasm, respiratory failure, dyspnea, nasal congestion, cough. *Gastrointestinal*: nausea, diarrhea, dyspepsia, anorexia. *Systemic*: including dry mouth; angioedema; urticaria; rash; depression; increase in signs and symptoms of myasthenia gravis; paresthesia; somnolence; insomnia; nightmares; behavioral changes; psychic disturbances, including confusion, hallucinations, anxiety, disorientation, nervousness; asthenia/fatigue and chest pain; alopecia and psoriasiform rash or exacerbation of psoriasis; systemic lupus erythematosus; retroperitoneal fibrosis; decreased libido; impotence; Peyronie's disease.

Pregnancy Category C.

Drug Interactions Because of the potential for serious adverse reactions in nursing infants, a decision should be made whether to discontinue nursing or to discontinue the drug, taking into account the importance of the drug to the mother. Safety and efficacy in pediatric patients have not been established.

Tissue Plasminogen Activator

Brand Name   Alteplase (off-label).

Class of Drug   Tissue plasminogen activator produced by recombinant DNA technology.

Indications   Experimental: tissue plasminogen activator (TPA) and gas tamponade for subretinal central hemorrhage; treatment of fibrinous reaction after surgery.

Dosage Form   Solution for intraocular use 500 U/μg.

Dose   *Fibrinous reaction after surgery*: 1,500–12,500 U. *Subretinal central hemorrhage*: 2,500–12,500 U

Contraindications   In patients hypersensitive to the product or any of its components.

Adverse Reactions   Most common complication is bleeding.

Pregnancy Category   C.

Drug Interactions   It is not known whether this drug is excreted in human milk. Safety and effectiveness in pediatric patients have not been established.

Tobramycin

Brand Name	AK-Tob; Tobrex; Tobrasol; TobraDex.
Class of Drug	Antibiotic.
Indications	Topical treatment of superficial infections of the external eye and adnexa; such as conjunctivitis; keratitis blepharitis; dacryocystitis; staphylococci, including *S. aureus* and *S. epidermidis* (coagulase-positive and coagulase-negative) and including penicillin-resistant strains; streptococci, including some of the group A beta-hemolytic species, some nonhemolytic species, and some *S. pneumoniae*; *P. aeruginosa*; *E. coli*; *K. pneumoniae*; *E. aerogenes*; *P. mirabilis*; *M. morganii*; most *P. vulgaris* strains; *H. influenzae* and *H. aegyptius*; *M. lacunata*; *A. calcoaceticus*; some *Neisseria* spp.
Dosage Form	Topical ophthalmic drops. Topical ophthalmic ointment.
Dose	1–2 drops every 4 h.
Contraindications	In patients hypersensitive to the product or any of its components.
Warnings	Not for injection into the eye. Cross-sensitivity to other aminoglycoside antibiotics may occur.
Adverse Reactions	Hypersensitivity and localized ocular toxicity, including lid itching and swelling, and conjunctival erythema.
Pregnancy Category	C.
Drug Interactions	It is not known whether this drug is excreted in human milk. Safety and effectiveness in pediatric patients younger than 2 years of age have not been established.

Travoprost

Brand Name	Travatan.
Class of Drug	Synthetic prostaglandin F-2 (alpha) analogue.
Indications	For the reduction of elevated IOP in patients with OAG or ocular hypertension who are intolerant of other IOP-lowering medications or insufficiently responsive to another IOP-lowering medication.
Dosage Form	Topical ophthalmic drops: travoprost ophthalmic solution 0.004%.
Dose	1 drop once per day in the evening.
Contraindications	In patients with known hypersensitivity to the product or any of its components or to benzalkonium chloride. Should be used with caution in patients with a history of intraocular inflammation (iritis/uveitis), and should generally not be used

in patients with active intraocular inflammation. Macular edema, including cystoid macular edema, has been reported during treatment with prostaglandin F-2 (alpha) analogues. These reports have mainly occurred in aphakic patients, pseudophakic patients with a torn posterior lens capsule, or patients with known risk factors for macular edema. Solution should be used with caution in these patients.

Adverse Reactions *Most frequent*: Ocular—ocular hyperemia, increased pigmentation of the iris and periorbital tissue, increased pigmentation and growth of eyelashes; these changes may be permanent. Decreased visual acuity, eye discomfort, foreign-body sensation, pain, pruritus, abnormal vision, blepharitis, blurred vision, cataract, cells, conjunctivitis, dry eye, eye disorder, flare, iris discoloration, keratitis, lid-margin crusting, photophobia, subconjunctival hemorrhage, tearing, angina pectoris. Nonocular—anxiety, arthritis, back pain, bradycardia, bronchitis, cold syndrome, depression, dyspepsia, gastrointestinal disorder, headache, hypercholesterolemia, hypertension, hypotension, infection, pain, prostate disorder, sinusitis, urinary incontinence, UTI.

Warnings Has been reported to cause changes to pigmented tissues: The most frequently reported have been increased pigmentation of the iris and periorbital tissue (eyelid) and increased pigmentation and growth of eyelashes. These changes may be permanent

Pregnancy Category C.

Drug Interactions It is not known whether this drug or its metabolites are excreted in human milk. Safety and effectiveness in pediatric patients have not been established.

Trifluridine

Brand Name Viroptic.

Class of Drug Antiviral.

Indications Indicated for the treatment of primary keratoconjunctivitis and recurrent epithelial keratitis due to herpes simplex virus types 1 and 2.

Dosage Form Topical ophthalmic solution 1%.

Dose 1 drop onto the cornea of affected eye(s) every 2 h while awake for a maximum daily dosage of 9 drops until the corneal ulcer has completely re-epithelialized. Following re-epithelialization, treatment for an additional 7 days of 1 drop every 4 h while awake for a minimum daily dosage of 5 drops is recommended. If there are no signs of improvement after 7 days of therapy or complete re-epithelialization has not occurred after 14 days of therapy, other forms of therapy should be considered. Continuous administration for periods exceeding 21 days should be avoided because of potential ocular toxicity.

Contraindications In patients who develop hypersensitivity reactions or chemical intolerance to the product or any of its components.

Warnings Recommended dosage and frequency of administration should not be exceeded. It should be prescribed only for patients who have a clinical diagnosis of herpetic keratitis.

Adverse Reactions Mild, transient burning or stinging, palpebral edema, superficial punctate keratopathy, epithelial keratopathy, hypersensitivity reaction, stromal edema, irritation, keratitis sicca, hyperemia, and increased IOP.

Trimethoprim Sulfate

Brand Name Polytrim; Polymyxin B Sulfate; Trimethoprim Sulfate.

Class of Drug Synthetic antibiotic. Blocks the production of tetrahydrofolic acid from dihydrofolic acid by binding to and reversibly inhibiting the enzyme dihydrofolate reductase. This binding is stronger for the bacterial enzyme than for the corresponding mammalian enzyme and therefore selectively interferes with bacterial biosynthesis of nucleic acids and proteins.

Indications In the treatment of surface ocular bacterial infections, including acute bacterial conjunctivitis, and blepharoconjunctivitis caused by susceptible strains of the following microorganisms: *S. aureus, S. epidermidis, S. pyogenes, S. faecalis, S. pneumoniae, H. influenzae, H. aegyptius, E. coli, K. pneumoniae, P. mirabilis, P. vulgaris, E. aerogenes*, and *S. marcescens*.

Dosage Form Topical ophthalmic drops.

Dose 1 drop every 3 h (maximum of six doses per day).

Contraindications As a prophylaxis or treatment of ophthalmia neonatorum.

Warnings Not for injection into the eye.

Adverse Reactions Increased redness, burning, stinging, and/or itching; lid edema; tearing; and/or circumocular rash.

Pregnancy Category C.

Drug Interactions It is not known whether this drug is excreted in human milk. Safety and effectiveness in children younger than 2 months of age have not been established.

Tropicamide

Brand Name	Mydriacyl; Opticyl.
Class of Drug	Cycloplegic, mydriatic.
Indications	Dilation of the pupil; used before eye examinations, such as cycloplegic refraction and examination of the fundus of the eye. May also be used before and after surgery.
Dosage Form	Topical ophthalmic drops, tropicamide solution 0.5, 1%.
Dose	*Cycloplegic refraction*: Adults—1 drop of 1% solution, repeated once in 5 min. Children—1 drop of 0.5–1% solution, repeated once in 5 min. *Fundus examination*: Adults and children—1 drop of 0.5% solution 15–20 min before examination.
Contraindications	In patients with a known hypersensitivity to the product or any of its components.
Warnings	Infants and young children and children with blond hair or blue eyes may be especially sensitive to the effects of tropicamide. This may increase the chance or severity of some of the side effects during treatment. May worsen brain damage (in children), Down syndrome (in children and adults), or glaucoma or spastic paralysis (in children).
Adverse Reactions	Light sensitivity; stinging; blurred vision; headache, clumsiness, unsteadiness; confusion; fast heartbeat; flushing or redness of face; hallucinations; increased thirst or dryness of mouth; skin rash; slurred speech; swollen stomach in infants; unusual behavior, especially in children; unusual drowsiness, tiredness, or weakness.
Pregnancy Category	C.
Drug Interactions	Studies on effects in pregnancy have not been done; has not been reported to cause problems in nursing babies.

Trypan Blue

Brand Name	Vision Blue.
Class of Drug	Stain.
Dosage Form	Solution.
Dose	For inner-limiting membrane staining:*After pars plana vitrectomy and induction of posterior vitreous detachment*: 0.5 ml trypan blue 0.06% in phosphate-buffered saline (PBS) injected over the posterior pole in an air-filled eye. *For lens capsule staining*: 0.5 ml trypan blue 0.06% in PBS injected over the anterior capsule in an air-filled anterior chamber.
Warnings	Contains chemical known to cause cancer.

Unoprostone Isopropyl

Brand Name   Rescula.

Class of Drug   Glaucoma. Prostaglandin analog.

Indications   For the reduction of elevated IOP in patients with OAG or ocular hypertension who are intolerant of or insufficiently responsive to another IOP-lowering medication.

Dosage Form   Topical ophthalmic drops: unoprostone isopropyl ophthalmic solution 0.15%.

Dose   1 drop two times per day.

Contraindications   In patients with a known hypersensitivity to unoprostone isopropyl, benzalkonium chloride, or any other components of this product. Should be used with caution in patients with active intraocular inflammation (e.g., uveitis).

Warnings   Has been reported to cause changes to pigmented tissue; these changes may be permanent.

Adverse Reactions   Ocular: burning, stinging, dry eyes, itching, increased length of eyelashes, and conjunctival injection (hyperemia), abnormal vision, eyelid disorder, foreign-body sensation, lacrimation disorder, blepharitis, cataract, conjunctivitis, corneal lesion, discharge from the eye, eye hemorrhage, eye pain, keratitis, irritation, photophobia, vitreous disorder, acute elevated IOP, color blindness, corneal deposits, corneal edema, corneal opacity, diplopia, hyperpigmentation of the eyelid, increased number of eyelashes, iris hyperpigmentation, iritis, optic atrophy, ptosis, retinal hemorrhage, visual-field defect. Nonocular: flu-like syndrome, allergic reaction, back pain, bronchitis, cough, dizziness, headache, hypertension, insomnia, pharyngitis, pain, rhinitis.

Pregnancy Category   C.

Drug Interactions   It is not known whether topical ocular administration could result in sufficient systemic absorption to produce detectable quantities in human milk. Safety and effectiveness in pediatric patients have not been established.

Valacyclovir

Brand Name   Valtrex.
Class of Drug   Antiviral.
Indications   Herpes zoster (shingles), treatment or suppression of genital herpes in immunocompetent individuals, suppression of recurrent genital herpes in HIV-infected individuals, cold sores (herpes labialis).
Dosage Form   Oral.
Dose   *Herpes zoster*: 1 g orally three times per day for 7 days; initiate therapy at the earliest signs or symptoms and is most effective when started within 48 h of the onset of zoster rash. *Genital herpes*: Initial episode—1 g two times per day for 10 days; most effective when administered within 48 h of the onset of the earliest signs or symptoms. Recurrent episodes—500 mg two times per day for 3 days; initiate therapy at the first signs or symptoms of an episode. Suppressive therapy—1 g once per day in patients with normal immune function. In patients with a history of nine or fewer recurrences per year, an alternative dose is 500 mg once per day. Safety and efficacy beyond 1 year have not been established. In HIV-infected patients with CD4 cell count ≥100 cells/mm^3, recommended dosage for chronic suppressive therapy of recurrent genital herpes is 500 mg two times per day. Safety and efficacy beyond 6 months in patients with HIV infection have not been established. *Cold sores (herpes labialis)*: 2 g two times per day for 1 day taken about 12 h apart; initiate therapy at the earliest signs or symptoms (e.g., tingling, itching, burning).
                        In patients with reduced renal function, reduction in dosage is recommended. Patients requiring hemodialysis should receive the recommended dose after hemodialysis. Supplemental doses should not be required following chronic ambulatory peritoneal dialysis and continuous arteriovenous hemofiltration/dialysis.
Contraindications   In patients with a known hypersensitivity or intolerance to the product or any of its components or to acyclovir.
Warnings   TTP/HUS, in some cases resulting in death, has occurred in patients with advanced HIV disease and also in allogeneic bone marrow transplant and renal transplant recipients participating in clinical trials at doses of 8 g per day. Acute renal failure and central nervous system symptoms have been reported in patients with underlying renal disease who have received inappropriately high doses for their level of renal function. Similar caution should be exercised when administering to geriatric patients and patients receiving potentially nephrotoxic agents.
Adverse Reactions   *General*: headache, fatigue, dizziness, facial edema, hypertension, tachycardia. *Allergic*: acute hypersensitivity reactions, including anaphylaxis, angioedema, dyspnea, pruritus, rash, urticaria. *CNS*: aggressive behavior; agitation; ataxia; coma;

confusion; depression; decreased consciousness; dysarthria; encephalopathy; mania; psychosis, including auditory and visual hallucinations; seizures, tremors. *Ocular*: visual abnormalities. *Gastrointestinal*: nausea, vomiting, abdominal pain, diarrhea. *Hepatobiliary tract and pancreas*: liver enzyme abnormalities, hepatitis. *Renal*: elevated creatinine, renal failure. *Hematologic*: thrombocytopenia, aplastic anemia, leukocytoclastic vasculitis, TTP/HUS. *Skin*: erythema multiforme; rashes, including photosensitivity; alopecia. *Renal impairment*: renal failure and CNS symptoms have been reported in patients with renal impairment who received Valtrex or acyclovir at greater than the recommended dose; dose reduction is recommended in this patient population. *Others*: dysmenorrhea, arthralgia. *Laboratory abnormalities*: elevated alkaline phosphatase, ALT, AST; decreased neutrophil, platelet counts.

Pregnancy Category   C.

Drug Interactions   No dosage adjustment is recommended when coadministered with digoxin, antacids, thiazide diuretics, cimetidine, or probenecid in subjects with normal renal function..

Valganciclovir

Brand Name   Valcyte Tablets.

Class of Drug   Antiviral.

Indications   For CMV retinitis in patients with AIDS; prevention of CMV disease in kidney, heart, and kidney–pancreas transplant patients at high risk [donor CMV seropositive/recipient CMV seronegative (D+/R-)]. Safety and efficacy for prevention of CMV disease in other solid organ transplant patients, such as lung transplant patients, have not been established.

Dosage Form   Oral tablet.

Dose   Valcyte tablets cannot be substituted for Cytovene capsules on a one-to-one basis. Dosage and administration as described below should be closely followed. *Treatment of CMV retinitis*: Induction—900 mg (2, 450 mg tablets) two times per day for 21 days with food. Maintenance—following induction treatment, or in patients with inactive CMV retinitis, 900 mg (2, 450 mg tablets) once per day with food. *Prevention of CMV disease in heart, kidney, and kidney–pancreas transplantation*: 900 mg (2, 450 mg tablets) once per day with food, starting within 10 days of transplantation until 100 days posttransplantation.

Serum creatinine or CrCl levels should be monitored carefully. Dosage adjustment is required according to CrCl. Increased

Contraindications
monitoring for cytopenias may be warranted in patients with renal impairment.
In patients with hypersensitivity to the product or any of its components or to ganciclovir. Should not be administered if the absolute neutrophil count is less than 500 cells/μl, platelet count is less than 25,000/μl, or hemoglobin is less than 8 g/dl. Should not be prescribed to patients receiving hemodialysis; for patients on hemodialysis (CrCl <10 ml/min), a dose recommendation cannot be given.

Warnings
Clinical toxicity of Valcyte, which is metabolized to ganciclovir, includes granulocytopenia, anemia, and thrombocytopenia. In animal studies, ganciclovir was carcinogenic, teratogenic, and caused aspermatogenesis. Valcyte tablets should, therefore, be used with caution in patients with preexisting cytopenias or who have received or who are receiving myelosuppressive drugs or irradiation. Should be considered a potential teratogen and carcinogen in humans with the potential to cause birth defects and cancers. Women of childbearing potential should be advised to use effective contraception during treatment. Similarly, men should be advised to practice barrier contraception during, and for at least 90 days following, treatment. Not indicated for use in liver transplant patients. In liver transplant patients, there was a significantly higher incidence of tissue-invasive CMV disease in the Valcyte-treated group compared with the oral ganciclovir group.

Adverse Reactions
Valganciclovir, a prodrug of ganciclovir, is rapidly converted to ganciclovir after oral administration. Adverse events known to be associated with ganciclovir usage can therefore be expected to occur.

Pregnancy Category
C.

Drug Interactions
Because the drug is rapidly and extensively converted to ganciclovir, interactions associated with ganciclovir will be expected. Zidovudine and valganciclovir each have the potential to cause neutropenia and anemia. Some patients may not tolerate concomitant therapy at full dosage. Patients taking probenecid concomitantly should be monitored for evidence of ganciclovir toxicity. Patients with renal impairment on concomitant mycophenolate mofetil should be monitored carefully, as levels of metabolites of both drugs may increase. Patients on concomitant didanosine should be closely monitored for didanosine toxicity.

Vancomycin Hydrochloride

Brand Name	Vancocin.
Class of Drug	Antibiotic.
Indications	In the treatment of enterocolitis caused by *S. aureus* (including methicillin-resistant strains) and antibiotic-associated pseudomembranous colitis caused by *C. difficile*. Parenteral administration is not effective for the above indications; therefore, it must be given orally for these indications. Orally administered, it is not effective for other types of infection.
Dosage Form	Oral; injectable.
Dose	*Adults*: Used in treating antibiotic-associated pseudomembranous colitis caused by *C. difficile* and staphylococcal enterocolitis; is not effective by the oral route for other types of infections. Usual adult total daily dosage is 500 mg to 2 g administered orally in 3 or 4 divided doses for 7–10 days. *Pediatric patients*: Usual daily dosage is 40 mg/kg in 3 or 4 divided doses for 7–10 days. Total daily dosage should not exceed 2 g.
Contraindications	In patients with a known hypersensitivity to this antibiotic or any of its components.
Warnings	Some patients with inflammatory disorders of the intestinal mucosa may have significant systemic absorption and, therefore, may be at risk for the development of adverse reactions associated with the parenteral administration. The risk is greater if renal impairment is present. It should be noted that the total systemic and renal clearances are reduced in the elderly. Monitoring serum concentrations may be appropriate in some instances, e.g., in patients with renal insufficiency.
Adverse Reactions	*Nephrotoxicity*: rarely, renal failure—principally manifested by increased serum creatinine or BUN concentrations, especially in patients given large doses of i.v.-administered vancomycin—has been reported. Rare cases of interstitial nephritis have been reported; most of these have occurred in patients who were given aminoglycosides concomitantly or who had preexisting kidney dysfunction. When vancomycin was discontinued, azotemia resolved in most patients. *Ototoxicity*: A few dozen cases of hearing loss associated with i.v.-administered vancomycin have been reported; most of these patients had kidney dysfunction or a preexisting hearing loss or were receiving concomitant treatment with an ototoxic drug. Vertigo, dizziness, and tinnitus have been reported rarely. *Hematopoietic*: Reversible neutropenia, usually starting 1 week or more after onset of i.v. therapy or after a total dose of more than 25 g has been reported for several dozen patients. Neutropenia appears to be promptly reversible when vancomycin is discontinued. Thrombocytopenia has rarely

been reported. *Miscellaneous*: infrequently; anaphylaxis, drug fever, chills, nausea, eosinophilia, rashes (including exfoliative dermatitis), Stevens–Johnson syndrome, toxic epidermal necrolysis, and rare cases of vasculitis have been reported.

Pregnancy Category   B.

Drug Interactions   Excreted in human milk based on information obtained with i.v. administration. However, systemic absorption is very low following oral administration. It is not known whether oral vancomycin is excreted in human milk, as no studies following oral administration have been done. Safety and effectiveness in pediatric patients have not been established.

Verteporfin

Brand Name   Visudyne.

Class of Drug   Light sensitizer, light-activated; used in photodynamic therapy.

Indications   For the treatment of patients with predominantly classic subfoveal choroidal neovascularization due to AMD, pathologic myopia, or presumed ocular histoplasmosis (for other forms of CNV, just experimental).

Dosage Form   Solution for i.v. injection: each milliliter contains 2 mg verteporfin.

Dose   Reconstitute each vial with 7 ml sterile water for injection to provide 7.5 ml containing 2 mg/ml. Reconstituted Visudyne must be protected from light and used within 4 h. It is recommended that reconstituted Visudyne be inspected visually for particulate matter and discoloration prior to administration. The volume of reconstituted Visudyne required to achieve the desired dose of 6 mg/m^2 body surface area is withdrawn from the vial and diluted with 5% dextrose for injection to a total infusion volume of 30 ml. The full infusion volume is administered i.v. over 10 min at a rate of 3 ml/min using an appropriate syringe pump and in-line filter.

Contraindications   In patients with porphyria or a known hypersensitivity to the product or any of its components. Should be considered carefully in patients with moderate to severe hepatic impairment or biliary obstruction since there is no clinical experience in such patients.

Warnings   Following injection, care should be taken to avoid exposure of skin or eyes to direct sunlight or bright indoor light for 5 days. In the event of extravasation during infusion, the extravasation area must be thoroughly protected from direct light until swelling and discoloration have faded in order to prevent the occurrence of a local burn, which could be severe. If emergency surgery is necessary within 48 h after treatment, as much of the internal tissue as possible should be protected from intense light.

Adverse Reactions Injection site reactions (including extravasation and rashes) and visual disturbances (including blurred vision, decreased visual acuity, and visual field defects).*Ocular treatment site*: blepharitis, cataracts, conjunctivitis/conjunctival injection, dry eyes, ocular itching, severe vision loss with or without subretinal or vitreous hemorrhage, retinal or choroidal vessel nonperfusion. *Body as a whole*: asthenia, back pain (primarily during infusion), fever, flu syndrome, photosensitivity reactions. *Cardiovascular*: atrial fibrillation, hypertension, peripheral vascular disorder, *Dermatologic*: eczema. *Digestive*: constipation, gastrointestinal cancers, nausea. *Hemic and lymphatic*: anemia, decreased/increased WBC. *Hepatic* elevated LFTs. *Metabolic*: albuminuria, increased creatinine. *Musculoskeletal*: arthralgia, arthrosis, myasthenia. *Nervous system*: hypesthesia, sleep disorders, vertigo. *Respiratory*: cough, pharyngitis, pneumonia. *Special senses*: decreased hearing, diplopia. *Urogenital*: prostatic disorder.

Pregnancy Category C.

Drug Interactions It is not known whether verteporfin for injection is excreted in human milk. Safety and effectiveness in pediatric patients have not been established.

Vitamins with Minerals

Brand Name See following for details on specific supplements.

Class of Drug Vitamin and mineral supplement.

Indications Extensive intermediate size drusen, at least one large druse, noncentral geographic atrophy in one or both eyes, or advanced AMD or vision loss due to AMD in one eye.

Dosage Form Oral tablet.

Dose 1 tablet one or two times per day.

Warnings Risk for lung cancer associated with smoking and using beta-carotene. Adverse effects and toxicity over a long-term period are not known. Individual effects of each supplement are not known. Nutritional supplements can help some patients but will not protect all patients from advanced AMD because AMD is multifactorial in nature. Some patients receiving the study medication continued to progress to advanced AMD and lose vision over time. Vitamin A (beta-carotene) may be harmful in smokers and lead to increased cancer risk.

Adverse Reactions Trials suggest Vitamin A (beta-carotene) might be harmful in smokers and lead to an increased cancer risk; alcohol consumption may be associated with an increased risk of adverse effects. There is also concern that long-term use of vitamin A in high does (>5,000 IU per day) can increase the risk of osteoporosis in women;beta-carotene may cause orange stools and cause diarrhea or loose stools at onset of therapy that tend to resolve with continued use. Vitamin C and E may interfere with effectiveness of statin therapy. Elevated levels of zinc have been associated with neurodegeneration in animal models, elevation of glycosylated hemoglobin levels in type I diabetics, decreased glucose tolerance in type II diabetes, and elevated serum zinc levels may be found in patients with Alzheimer's disease. Necrotizing enterocolitis may occur when large doses of vitamin E are given. Withdrawal of chronic, high levels of vitamin C may lead to rebound deficiency due to increased clearance; probably requires taper or reduced dose at US MDR; prolonged high doses may cause renal calculi, especially in diabetics.

Pregnancy Category   Taking large amounts of a dietary supplements in pregnancy may be harmful to the mother and/or fetus and should be avoided.

Brand Name   ICaps.
Dosage Form   Vitamin A 14,320 IU 286%, vitamin C 226 mg 376%, vitamin E 200 IU 666%, zinc 34.8 mg 232%, copper 0.8 mg 40%.
Contraindications   *Most significant*: Wilson's disease. *Significant*: biliary tract disorder, copper deficiency. *Possibly significant:* liver disease.
Adverse Reactions   *Most frequent*: carotenodermia. *Rare*: abdominal pain with cramps, arthralgia, diarrhea, dizziness, dyspepsia, ecchymosis, gastrointestinal disorder, leukopenia, nausea, neutropenia, sideroblastic anemia.

Brand Name   Ocuvite.
Dosage Form   Vitamin A 1,000 IU 20% vitamin C 200 mg 330%, vitamin E 60 IU 200%, zinc 40 mg 270%, selenium 55 mcg 80%, copper 2 mg 100%, lutein 2 mg N/A.
Adverse Reactions   *Most frequent*: carotenodermia. *Rare*: arthralgia, diarrhea, dizziness, ecchymosis.

Brand Name   Ocuvite Extra.
Dosage Form   Vitamin A 1,000 IU 20%, vitamin C 300 mg 500%, vitamin E 100 IU 330%, riboflavin 3 mg 180%, niacinamide 40 mg 200%, zinc 40 mg 270%, selenium 55 mcg 80%, copper 2 mg 100%, manganese 5 mg 250%, L-glutathione 5 mg N/A, lutein 2 mg N/A.
Adverse Reactions   *Less frequent*: nausea, vomiting.

Brand Name   Ocuvite PreserVision.
Dosage Form   Beta-carotene 17.2 mg N/A, vitamin C 452 mg 753%, vitamin E 268 mg 2,680%, zinc 69.6 mg 464%, copper 1.6 mg N/A.

Contraindications	*Most significant*: Wilson's disease. *Significant*: biliary tract disorder, copper deficiency. *Possibly significant*: liver disease.
Adverse Reactions	*Most frequent*: carotenodermia. *Rare*: abdominal pain with cramps, arthralgia, diarrhea, dizziness, dyspepsia, ecchymosis, gastrointestinal disorder, leukopenia, nausea, neutropenia, sideroblastic anemia.

Brand Name	Ocuvite Lutein.
Dosage Form	Vitamin C 60 mg 100%, vitamin E 30 IU 100%, zinc 15 mg 100%, copper 2 mg 100%, lutein 6 mg N/A.
Contraindications	*Most significant*: hemolytic anemia from pyruvate kinase and G6PD deficiencies. *Possibly significant*: hemochromatosis, hyperoxaluria, hypoprothrombinemia due to vitamin K deficiency, renal calculi, sickle cell disease anemia, sideroblastic anemia, thalassemia anemia, type 1 diabetes mellitus, type 2 diabetes mellitus.
Adverse Reactions	*Rare*: abdominal pain with cramps, blurred vision, diarrhea, dizziness, erythema, fatigue, flushing, headache, increased urinary frequency, nausea, renal calculi, vomiting.
Drug Interactions	*Only when necessary*: in familial defective apolipoprotein B (FDB); category C in Briggs if dose exceeds recommended daily amount (RDA). *Lactation*: No known risk—no documented problems in humans; no documented problems with normal intake. *Pediatric*: Warning—no documented problems in children with normal intake.

Brand Name	Copper.
Indications	Component of enzymes in iron metabolism.
Dosage Form	*Oral*: as mineral supplements. *Injectable*: as trace minerals for TRN supplement.
Contraindications	Should be avoided in patients with biliary tract obstruction or Wilson's disease. May cause high blood levels of copper in patients with biliary disease or liver disease.
Adverse Reactions	Gastrointestinal distress, liver damage.
Pregnancy Category	C.
Drug Interactions	Absorption of copper decreases in the concurrent use of high doses of zinc or vitamin C.

Brand Name	Lutein.
Indications	Oxygenated carotinoid that forms the macular pigment, absorbs short wavelength of light, and quenches free radicals.
Dosage Form	Oral
Contraindications	Documented hypersensitivity.
Pregnancy Category	C.

Brand Name	Manganese.
Indications	Involved in the formation of bone as well as in enzymes involved in amino acid, cholesterol, and carbohydrate metabolism.
Dosage Form	*Oral*: as mineral supplements. *Injectable*: as trace minerals for TRN supplement.

Contraindications	Documented hypersensitivity.
Warnings	Eliminated via the bile; accumulates in patients with severe liver dysfunction and/or biliary tract obstruction.
Adverse Reactions	Elevated blood concentration and neurotoxicity.
Pregnancy Category	C.

Brand Name	Niacinamide.
Indications	Coenzyme or cosubstrate in many biological reduction or oxidation reactions; thus required for energy metabolism.
Dosage Form	Oral and injectable.
Contraindications	In insulin-dependent diabetes, aggravates blood sugar problems.
Adverse Reactions	*With injection only*: skin rash or itching; wheezing. *With prolonged use of extended-release niacin*: darkening of urine; light-gray-colored stools; loss of appetite; severe stomach pain; yellow eyes or skin. *Less common with niacin only*: feeling of warmth; flushing or redness of skin, especially on face and neck; headache. *With high doses*: Diarrhea; dizziness or faintness; dryness of skin; fever; frequent urination; itching of skin; joint pain; muscle aching or cramping; nausea or vomiting; side, lower back, or stomach pain; swelling of feet or lower legs; unusual thirst; unusual tiredness or weakness; unusually fast, slow, or irregular heartbeat.
Pregnancy Category	C.

Brand Name	Riboflavin (vitamin B2).
Indications	Coenzyme in numerous redox reactions.
Dosage Form	Oral.
Contraindications	In patients with known hypersensitivity to the product.
Adverse Reactions	May cause urine to become yellow-orange color; this effect is harmless.

Brand Name	Selenium.
Indications	Defense against oxidative stress and regulation of thyroid hormone action; reduction and oxidation status of vitamin C and other molecules.
Dosage Form	*Oral*: as mineral supplements. *Injectable*: as trace minerals for TRN supplement.
Warnings	Eliminated in urine and feces; may be adjusted, reduced, or omitted in renal dysfunction and/or gastrointestinal malfunction. In patients receiving blood transfusions, contribution from such transfusions should also be considered. Frequent selenium plasma level determinations are suggested as a guideline. Presence in placenta and umbilical cord blood has been reported in humans.
Adverse Reactions	Hair and nail brittleness and loss.
Pregnancy Category	C.
Drug Interactions	In animals, has been reported to enhance the action of vitamin E and decrease toxicity of mercury, cadmium, and arsenic.

Brand Name	Vitamin A.
Indications	Required for normal vision, gene expression, reproduction, embryonic development, and immune function.
Dosage Form	Oral.
Contraindications	In patients with documented hypersensitivity; hepatic insufficiency.
Warnings	Toxicity reported for chronic doses greater than 25,000 IU; caution if taking with other hepatotoxic medications and normal dietary amounts of beta-carotene.
Adverse Reactions	Teratological effects, liver toxicity.
Pregnancy Category	A; but X if dose exceeds RDA.

Brand Name	Vitamin C.
Indications	Cofactor for reactions requiring reduced copper or iron metalloenzyme and as a protective antioxidant.
Dosage Form	Oral.
Contraindications	In pregnancy in large doses.
Warnings	Withdrawal of chronic, high levels may lead to rebound deficiency due to increased clearance; probably requires taper or reduced dose. Prolonged high doses may cause renal calculi, especially in diabetics.
Adverse Reactions	Gastrointestinal disturbances, kidney stones, excess iron absorption.
Pregnancy Category	C.
Drug Interactions	Decreases effects of warfarin and fluphenazine; increases aspirin levels.

Brand Name	Vitamin E.
Indications	A metabolic function has not yet been identified. Its major function appears to be as a nonspecific, chain-breaking antioxidant.
Dosage Form	Oral.
Dose	Up to 800 IU per day.
Adverse Reactions	Hemorrhagic toxicity. Appears to be safe when consumed in amounts up to 1,000 IU a day although diarrhea and headaches have been reported. Doses of over 800 IU per day may interfere with the body's ability to clot blood, posing a risk to people taking blood thinners (anticoagulants).
Drug Interactions	May intensify blood-thinning effect of dalteparin, enoxaparin, or warfarin. High doses may inhibit the absorption of vitamin A.

Brand Name	Zinc.
Indications	Component of multiple enzymes and proteins; involved in the regulation of gene expression.
Dosage Form	Oral.
Dose	Up to 40 mg. per day.
Warnings	Total daily intake (from supplements, foods, and other sources combined) should not surpass 150 mg per day.
Adverse Reactions	Reduced copper status, anemia. In amounts greater than 200 mg per day can cause nausea, vomiting, and diarrhea.

Even 100 mg per day in supplement form over long periods can result in problems, including lowered levels of high-density lipoprotein (HDL) (»good«) cholesterol and diminished immune-system function. An association between excessive zinc and Alzheimer's disease has been made.

Drug Interactions   Absorption of copper may be compromised by long-term (one month or more) ingestion of zinc. If taking iron supplements, avoid absorption problems by taking zinc 2 h after the iron. Because zinc may decrease absorption of the antibiotics tetracycline, doxycycline, and minocycline making them less effective, take at least 2 h after the antibiotic.

Voriconazole

Brand Name   VFEND: injection, tablets, oral suspension.
Class of Drug   Antifungal.
Indications   *Invasive aspergillosis*: in clinical trials, the majority of isolates recovered were *Aspergillus fumigatus*. Small number of cases of culture-proven disease due to *Aspergillus* spp. other than *A. fumigatus*. *Esophageal candidiasis*; serious fungal infections caused by *Scedosporium apiospermum* (asexual form of *Pseudallescheria boydii*) and *Fusarium* spp., including *Fusarium solani*, in patients intolerant of, or refractory to, other therapy.
Dosage Form   Injection, oral tablets, oral suspension.
Dose   *Loading dose regimen*: 6 mg/kg i.v. every 12 h (for the first 24 h). *Maintenance dose*: IV—4 mg/kg every 12 h. Oral*— 200 mg every 12 h. (*Patients who weigh 40 kg or more should receive an oral maintenance dose of 200 mg every 12 h. Adult patients who weigh less than 40 kg should receive an oral maintenance dose of 100 mg every 12 h. If patient response is inadequate, the oral maintenance dose may be increased from 200 mg every 12 h to 300 mg every 12 h. For adult patients weighing less than 40 kg, the oral maintenance dose may be increased from 100 mg every 12 h to 150 mg every 12 h. If patients are unable to tolerate treatment, reduce the i.v. maintenance dose to 3 mg/kg every 12 h and the oral maintenance dose by 50 mg steps to a minimum of 200 mg every 12 h; or to 100 mg every 12 h for adult patients weighing less than 40 kg.)
Contraindications *Coadministration with*: CYP3A4 substrates terfenadine, astemizole, cisapride, pimozide, or quinidine, as increased plasma concentrations of these drugs can lead to QT prolongation and rare occurrences of *torsade de pointes;* sirolimus, as VFEND significantly increases sirolimus concentrations in healthy subjects; rifampin, carbamazepine, and long-acting

barbiturates, as these drugs are likely to significantly decrease plasma voriconazole concentrations; ritonavir (400 mg every 12 h), as ritonavir (400 mg every 12 h) significantly decreases plasma voriconazole concentrations in healthy subjects; efavirenz, as efavirenz significantly decreases voriconazole plasma concentrations while VFEND also significantly increases efavirenz plasma concentrations; rifabutin, as VFEND significantly increases rifabutin plasma concentrations and rifabutin also significantly decreases voriconazole plasma concentrations; ergot alkaloids (ergotamine and dihydroergotamine), as VFEND may increase plasma concentration of ergot alkaloids, which may lead to ergotism.

Warnings

Visual disturbances: if treatment continues beyond 28 days, visual function, including visual acuity, visual field, and color perception should be monitored. *Hepatic toxicity*: In clinical trials, there have been uncommon cases of serious hepatic reactions during treatment (including clinical hepatitis, cholestasis, and fulminant hepatic failure, including fatalities). LFTs should be evaluated at the start of and during therapy. *Galactose intolerance*: tablets contain lactose and should not be given to patients with rare hereditary problems of galactose intolerance, Lapp lactase deficiency, or glucose-galactose malabsorption. *Precautions*: Some azoles, including voriconazole, have been associated with prolongation of the QT interval on the electrocardiogram. During clinical development and post-marketing surveillance, there have been rare cases of *torsade de pointes*. Should be administered with caution to patients with these potentially proarrhythmic conditions. Rigorous attempts to correct potassium, magnesium, and calcium should be made before starting voriconazole. If patients develop a rash, they should be monitored closely and consideration given to discontinuation of treatment. Recommended that patients avoid strong, direct sunlight during therapy. No information regarding cross-sensitivity between voriconazole and other azole antifungal agents. Caution should be used when prescribing to patients with hypersensitivity to other azoles.

Adverse Reactions

Most frequent: Visual disturbances, fever, rash, vomiting, nausea, diarrhea, headache, sepsis, peripheral edema, abdominal pain, and respiratory disorder. Treatment-related adverse events that most often lead to discontinuation of therapy are elevated LFTs, rash, and visual disturbances. Visual disturbances—common; include altered/enhanced visual perception, blurred vision, color vision change and/or photophobia. In a study in healthy volunteers investigating the effect of 28-day treatment with voriconazole on retinal function, voriconazole caused a decrease in the electroretinogram (ERG) waveform amplitude, decrease in the visual field, and alteration in color perception. Fourteen days after end of dosing, ERG, visual fields, and color perception returned to normal.

Dermatological reactions: Rashes; photosensitivity; rarely serious cutaneous reactions, including Stevens–Johnson syndrome; toxic epidermal necrolysis; erythema multiform. *Less frequent*: Refer to the *Physicians' Desk Reference* (PDR).

Pregnancy Category   D.

Drug Interactions   Can cause fetal harm when administered to a pregnant woman.

Zinc Sulfate

Brand Name	Visine AC; Clear Eyes ACR.
Class of Drug	Astringent.
Indications	Temporary relief of discomfort and dryness of the eye due to minor eye irritations.
Dosage Form	Topical ophthalmic drops: zinc sulfate 0.25%.
Dose	1 or 2 drops up to four times per day.
Contraindications	In patients with a known hypersensitivity to the product or any of its components.
Warnings	Because products containing zinc sulfate usually also contain other active ingredient that may results in pupillary dilation, this product should be avoid if patient has glaucoma, except under the direction of an ophthalmologist.
Adverse Reactions	Burning, stinging, pain, increased redness of the eye, tearing, blurred vision, headache, tremor, nausea, sweating, nervousness, dizziness, drowsiness.
Pregnancy Category	C.

Dosage Summary
for Anti-infectives

Antibiotics

Name	Amikacin sulfate.
Spectrum	*Staphylococcus, Neisseria, Escherichia coli, Klebsiella, Enterobacter, Serratia, Citrobacter, Proteus, Providencia, Pseudomonas aeruginosa, Brucella, Yersinia pestis, Francisella tularensis, Acinetobacter.*
Indications (Ocular Disease)	Conjunctivitis, keratitis, endophthalmitis, especially for atypical mycobacteria.
Topical	10–50 mg/ml up to q1h.
Subconjunctival	25–125 mg/0.5 ml.
Intravitreal	0.2–0.4 mg/0.1 ml.
Intravenous/Oral	5–15 mg/kg qd, i.v. divided into two to three doses.

Name	Ampicillin sodium.
Spectrum	Gram-positive bacteria: *Staphylococcus aureus* (beta-lactamase and non-beta-lactamase-producing), *Staphylococcus epidermidis* (beta-lactamase and non-beta-lactamase-producing), *Staphylococcus saprophyticus* (beta-lactamase and non-beta-lactamase-producing), *Streptococcus faecalis* (*Enterococcus*), *Streptococcus pneumoniae* (formerly *Diplococcus pneumoniae*), *Streptococcus pyogenes, Streptococcus viridans*. Gram-negative bacteria: *Haemophilus influenzae* (beta-lactamase and non-beta-lactamase-producing). *Moraxella* (*Branhamella*) *catarrhalis* (beta-lactamase and non-beta-lactamase-producing). *E. coli* (beta-lactamase and non-beta-lactamase-producing). *Klebsiella* spp. (all known strains are beta-lactamase-producing). *Proteus mirabilis* (beta-lactamase and non-beta-lactamase-producing). *Proteus vulgaris, Providencia rettgeri, Providencia stuartii, Morganella morganii,* and *Neisseria gonorrhoeae* (beta-lactamase and non-beta-lactamase-producing). Anaerobes: *Clostridium* spp.; *Peptococcus* spp.; *Peptostreptococcus* spp.; *Bacteroides* spp., including *B. fragilis*. These are not beta-lactamase-producing strains and, therefore, are susceptible to ampicillin alone.
Indications (Ocular Disease)	Preseptal (p.o.) or orbital (i.v.) cellulites; perioperative for mucocele resection (i.v.).
Topical	50 mg/ml.
Subconjunctival	50–150 mg/0.5 ml.
Intravitreal	500 µg/0.1 ml.
Intravenous/Oral	4–12 g qd, i.v. divided into four doses, 250–500 mg p.o., t.i.d.

Name	Bacitracin zinc.
Spectrum	Most gram-positive bacilli/cocci, including hemolytic streptococci.
Indications (Ocular Disease)	Conjunctivitis, keratitis.
Topical	500–10,000 U qd to q.i.d.
Subconjunctival	5.000 U/0.5 ml.

Intravitreal	500–1,000 U/0.1 ml.
Intravenous/Oral	N/A.

Name	Cefazolin sodium.
Spectrum	Gram-positive bacteria,*E. coli, Klebsiella pneumoniae, Staphylococcus* spp.
Indications (Ocular Disease)	Keratitis, corneal ulcer.
Topical	50 mg/ml up to q1h.
Subconjunctival	100 mg/0.5 ml.
Intravitreal	2.25 mg/0.1 ml.
Intravenous/Oral	50–100 mg/kg qd, i.v. divided into three to four doses.

Name	Ceftazidime.
Spectrum	Aerobic gram-negative:*Citrobacter* spp., including *C. freundii* and *C. diversus; Enterobacter* spp., including *E. cloacae* and *E. aerogenes; E. coli; H. influenzae*, including ampicillin-resistant strains; *Klebsiella* spp., including *K. pneumoniae; Neisseria meningitidis; P. mirabilis; P. vulgaris; Pseudomonas* spp., including *P. aeruginosa; Serratia* spp.
	Aerobic gram-positive: *S. aureus*, including penicillinase- and non-penicillinase-producing strains; *Streptococcus agalactiae* (group B streptococci); *S. pneumoniae; S. pyogenes* (group A beta-hemolytic streptococci).
	Anaerobic: *Bacteroides* spp. (Note: Many strains of *B. fragilis* are resistant.)
Indications (Ocular Disease)	Infectious cavernous sinus thrombosis (i.v.), open globe (topical + i.v.), endophthalmitis (all routes of administration).
Topical	50 mg/ml q1h.
Subconjunctival	100 mg/0.5 ml.
Intravitreal	1–2.25 mg/0.1 ml.
Intravenous/Oral	1–2 g i.v. q8h.

Name	Ceftriaxone.
Spectrum	Aerobic gram-negative microorganisms:*Acinetobacter calcoaceticus; E. aerogenes; E. cloacae; E. coli; H. influenzae*, including ampicillin-resistant and beta-lactamase-producing strains; *Haemophilus parainfluenzae; Klebsiella oxytoca; K. pneumoniae; Moraxella catarrhalis*, including beta-lactamase-producing strains; *M. morganii; N. gonorrhoeae*, including penicillinase- and non-penicillinase-producing strains; *N. meningitidis; P. mirabilis; P. vulgaris; Serratia marcescens*. Also active against many strains of *P. aeruginosa*. (Note: Many strains that are multiply resistant to other antibiotics, e.g., penicillins, cephalosporins, and aminoglycosides, are susceptible to ceftriaxone.)
	Aerobic gram-positive microorganisms: *S. aureus*, including penicillinase-producing strains; *S. epidermidis; S. pneumoniae; S. pyogenes*; viridans group streptococci. (Note: Methicillin-resistant staphylococci are resistant to cephalosporins, including ceftriaxone. Most strains of group D streptococci

and enterococci, e.g., *Enterococcus* (*Streptococcus*) *faecalis*, are resistant.)
Anaerobic microorganisms: *B. fragilis, Clostridium* spp., *Peptostreptococcus* spp. (Note: Most strains of *Clostridium difficile* are resistant.)

Indications (Ocular Disease)
Orbital cellulites (i.v.).

Topical — N/A.
Subconjunctival — 100 mg/0.5 ml.
Intravitreal — 3.0 mg/0.1 ml.
Intravenous/Oral — 2 g i.v., q12h.

Name — Clindamycin.
Spectrum — Aerobic gram-positive cocci, including:*S. aureus, S. epidermidis* (penicillinase and non-penicillinase-producing strains) (Note: When tested by in vitro methods, some staphylococcal strains originally resistant to erythromycin rapidly develop resistance to clindamycin; streptococci (except *S. faecalis*), pneumococci.)
Anaerobic gram-negative bacilli, including: *Bacteroides* spp., including *B. fragilis* group and *B. melaninogenicus* group; *Fusobacterium* spp.
Anaerobic gram-positive non-spore-forming bacilli, including: *Propionibacterium, Eubacterium, Actinomyces* spp.
Anaerobic and microaerophilic gram-positive cocci, including: *Peptococcus* spp., *Peptostreptococcus* spp., *Microaerophilic streptococci.*
Clostridia: Clostridia are more resistant than most anaerobes to clindamycin. Most *Clostridium perfringens* are susceptible but other species, e.g., *Clostridium sporogenes* and *Clostridium tertium*, are frequently resistant to clindamycin. Susceptibility testing should be done. Cross-resistance has been demonstrated between clindamycin and lincomycin. Antagonism has been demonstrated between clindamycin and erythromycin.

Indications (Ocular Disease)
Conjunctivitis, keratitis, toxoplasmosis.

Topical — 20–50 mg/ml up to q1h.
Subconjunctival — 15–50 mg/0.5 ml.
Intravitreal — 200 µg-1.0 mg/0.1 ml.
Intravenous/Oral — 300–600 mg p.o., q.i.d.

Name — Colistimethate sodium.
Spectrum — Aerobic gram-negative microorganisms:*E. aerogenes, E. coli, K. pneumoniae, P. aeruginosa.*
Indications (Ocular Disease) — Bacteria blepharitis, bacteria conjunctivitis.
Topical — 10 mg/ml.
Subconjunctival — 15–25 mg/0.5 ml.
Intravitreal — 100 mcg/0.1 ml.

Intravenous/Oral	2.5–5 mg/kg qd in two to four divided i.m. or i.v. doses for patients with normal renal function.
Name	Erythromycin.
Spectrum	Gram-positive organisms:*Corynebacterium diphtheriae, Corynebacterium minutissimum, Listeria monocytogenes, S. aureus* (resistant organisms may emerge during treatment), *S. pneumoniae, S. pyogenes.*
	Gram-negative organisms: *Bordetella pertussis, Legionella pneumophila, N. gonorrhoeae.*
	Other microorganisms: *Chlamydia trachomatis, Entamoeba histolytica, Mycoplasma pneumoniae, Treponema pallidum, Ureaplasma urealyticum.*
Indications	Ophthalmia neonatorum, prevention of neonatal ophthalmia,
(Ocular Disease)	superficial ocular infection, bacterial blepharitis, bacterial conjunctivitis, bacterial keratitis, bacterial keratoconjunctivitis, blepharoconjunctivitis, chlamydial conjunctivitis, meibomianitis, trachoma.
Topical	0.5% qd to q.i.d.
Subconjunctival	100 mg/0.5 ml.
Intravitreal	0.5 mg/0.1 ml.
Intravenous/Oral	750–2,000 mg/day p.o./i.v. divided into three to four doses.
Name	Gentamicin sulfate.
Spectrum	Gram-positive bacteria:*Staphylococcus* spp., Gram-negative bacteria.
Indications	Conjunctivitis, corneal ulcer, keratitis, endophthalmitis.
(Ocular Disease)	Acquired anophthalmia, open globe.
Topical	0.3% q.i.d.
Subconjunctival	20–40 mg/0.5 ml.
Intravitreal	0.1–0.15 mg/0.1 ml.
Intravenous/Oral	1.5–5 mg/kg qd, i.v. divided into one to three doses.
Name	Imipenem/Cilastatin sodium.
Spectrum	Gram-positive aerobes:*Enterococcus faecalis* (formerly *S. faecalis*) [Note: Imipenem is inactive in vitro against *Enterococcus faecium* (formerly *Streptococcus faecium*)]; *S. aureus*, including penicillinase-producing strains; *S. epidermidis*, including penicillinase-producing strains (Note: Methicillin-resistant staphylococci should be reported as resistant to imipenem); *S. agalactiae* (group B streptococci); *S. pneumoniae; S. pyogenes.* Gram-negative aerobes: *Acinetobacter* spp.; *Citrobacter* spp.; *Enterobacter* spp.; *E. coli; Gardnerella vaginalis; H. influenzae; H. parainfluenzae; Klebsiella* spp.; *M. morganii; P. vulgaris; P. rettgeri; P. aeruginosa* (Note: Imipenem is inactive in vitro against *Xanthomonas (Pseudomonas) maltophilia* and some strains of *Pseudomonas cepacia*); *Serratia* spp., including *S. marcescens.* Gram-positive anaerobes: *Bifidobacterium* spp., *Clostridium* spp., *Eubacterium* spp., *Peptococcus* spp., *Peptostreptococcus* spp., *Propionibacterium* spp.

Gram-negative anaerobes: *Bacteroides* spp., including *B. fragilis*; *Fusobacterium* spp.

Indications (Ocular Disease)	Conjunctivitis, keratitis, endophthalmitis.
Topical	50 mg/ml.
Subconjunctival	100 mg/0.5 ml.
Intravenous/Oral	1.5–4g qd, i.v. divided into three to four doses.

Name	Kanamycin sulfate.
Spectrum	Gram-negative bacteria, staphylococci, atypical mycobacteria.
Indications (Ocular Disease)	Corneal abrasion, keratitis, conjunctivitis.
Topical	10–20 g/ml q.i.d. to q4h.
Subconjunctival	10–20 g/0.5 ml.
Intravitreal	N/A.
Intravenous/Oral	0.5 g i.m., t.i.d.

Name	Neomycin sulfate.
Spectrum	Gram-positive:*S. aureus*, coagulase-negative staphylococci, *S. pyogenes, E. faecalis, Mycobacterium tuberculosis*. Gram-negative: *N. meningitidis, N. gonorrhoeae, H. influenzae, E. coli, K. pneumoniae*. Other: *Borrelia* spp., *Pasteurella* spp., *Vibrio* spp., *Leptospira* spp.
Indications (Ocular Disease)	Conjunctivitis, corneal ulcer, keratitits, acanthamoeba keratitis.
Topical	10–30 mg/ml q.i.d. to q2h.
Subconjunctival	100–500 mg/0.5 ml.
Intravitreal	N/A.
Intravenous/Oral	N/A.

Name	Penicillin G.
Spectrum	Staphylococci (except penicillinase-producing strains), streptococci (groups A, C, G, H, L, M), and pneumococci. Other organisms: *N. gonorrhoeae, C. diphtheriae, Bacillus anthracis, Clostridia* spp., *Actinomyces bovis/israelii, Streptobacillus moniliformis, L. monocytogenes*, and *Leptospira* spp. *Treponema pallidum* is extremely susceptible to the bactericidal action of penicillin G.
Indications (Ocular Disease)	Canaliculitis, infectious cavernous sinus thrombosis.
Topical	100,000 U/ml for irrigation.
Subconjunctival	500,000–1 million U/0.5 ml.
Intravitreal	1,000–5,000 U/0.1 ml.
Intravenous/Oral	12–24 million U qd, i.v. divided into four doses.

Name	Piperacillin.
Spectrum	Aerobic and facultatively anaerobic organisms. Gram-negative bacteria: *E. coli; P. mirabilis; P. vulgaris; M. morganii* (formerly *P. morganii*); *P. rettgeri* (formerly *Proteus*

rettgeri); *Serratia* spp., including *S. marcescens* and *Serratia liquefaciens*; *K. pneumoniae*; *Klebsiella* spp.; *Enterobacter* spp., including *E. aerogenes* and *E. cloacae*; *Citrobacter* spp., including *C. freundii* and *C. diversus*; *Salmonella* spp.; *Shigella* spp.; *P. aeruginosa*; *Pseudomonas* spp., including *P. cepacia, P. maltophilia*, and *Pseudomonas fluorescens*; *Acinetobacter* spp. (formerly Mima-Herellea); *H. influenzae* (non-beta-lactamase-producing strains); *N. gonorrhoeae; N. meningitidis; Moraxella* spp. (formerly *Pasteurella*).

Gram-positive bacteria: Group D streptococci, including, enterococci (*S. faecalis, S. faecium*), nonenterococci; beta-hemolytic streptococci, including, group A *Streptococcus* (*S. pyogenes*), group B *Streptococcus* (*S. agalactiae*); *S. pneumonia; S. viridans; S. aureus* (non-penicillinase-producing); *S. epidermidis* (non-penicillinase-producing).

Anaerobic bacteria: *Actinomyces* spp.; *Bacteroides* spp., including *B. fragilis* group (*B. fragilis, Bacteroides vulgatus*); non-*B. fragilis* group (*B. melaninogenicus*); *Bacteroides asaccharolyticus; Clostridium* spp., including, *C. perfringens* and *C. difficile; Eubacterium* spp.; *Fusobacterium* spp., including *F. nucleatum* and *F. necrophorum; Peptococcus* spp.; *Peptostreptococcus* spp.; *Veillonella* spp. (Piperacillin has been shown to be active in vitro against these organisms; however, clinical efficacy has not yet been established.)

Indications (Ocular Disease)	Ocular or periocular infection.
Topical	12.5 mg/ml.
Subconjunctival	100 mg/0.5 ml.
Intravenous/Oral	6–16 g qd, i.v. divided into three to four doses.

Name	Polymyxin B sulfate.
Spectrum	Gram-negative bacteria, especially *P. aeruginosa*.
Indications (Ocular Disease)	Conjunctivitis, corneal abrasion, keratitis.
Topical	5–10 mg/ml q.i.d. to q4h.
Subconjunctival	10–25 mg/0.5 ml.
Intravitreal	N/A.
Intravenous/Oral	75–100 mg p.o., q.i.d.; 1.5–2.5 mg/kg qd divided into three to four doses.

Name	Ticarcillin disodium.
Spectrum	Gram-positive aerobes: *S. aureus* (beta-lactamase and non-beta-lactamase-producing); *S. epidermidis* (beta-lactamase and non-beta-lactamase-producing) (Note: Staphylococci resistant to methicillin/oxacillin must be considered resistant to ticarcillin/clavulanic acid.)

Gram-negative aerobes: *Citrobacter* spp. (beta-lactamase and non-beta-lactamase-producing); *Enterobacter* spp., including *E. cloacae* (beta-lactamase and non-beta-lactamase-producing) (Note: Although most strains of *Enterobacter* spp. are resistant in vitro, clinical efficacy has been demonstrated in urinary tract and gynecologic infections caused by these organisms); *E. coli* (beta-lactamase and non-beta-lactamase-producing); *H. influenzae* (beta-lactamase and non-beta-lactamase-producing); *Klebsiella* spp., including *K. pneumoniae* (beta-lactamase and non-beta-lactamase-producing); *Pseudomonas* spp., including *P. aeruginosa* (beta-lactamase and non-beta-lactamase-producing); *S. marcescens* (beta-lactamase and non-beta-lactamase-producing)· (Note: beta-lactamase-negative ampicillin-resistant (BLNAR) strains of *H. influenzae* must be considered resistant to ticarcillin/clavulanic acid.)

Anaerobic bacteria: *B. fragilis* group (beta-lactamase and non-beta-lactamase-producing); *Prevotella* (formerly *Bacteroides*) *melaninogenicus* (beta-lactamase and non-beta-lactamase-producing).

Indications (Ocular Disease)	Ocular or periocular infection.
Topical	6 mg/ml.
Subconjunctival	100 mg/0.5 ml.
Intravenous/Oral	200–300 mg/kg qd, i.v. divided into three doses.

Name	Tobramycin sulfate.
Spectrum	Gram-positive:*Staphylococcus* spp. Gram-negative: especially *P. aeruginosa*.
Indications (Ocular Disease)	Corneal abrasion, keratitis, conjunctivitis.
Topical	0.3% q.i.d. to q1h.
Subconjunctival	20–40 mg/0.5 ml.
Intravitreal	0.2 mg/0.1 ml.
Intravenous/Oral	3–5 mg/kg qd, i.v. divided into one to three doses.

Name	Vancomycin hydrochloride.
Spectrum	Aerobic gram-positive:*S. aureus*, including methicillin-resistant strains) associated with enterocolitis. Anaerobic gram-positive: *C. difficile* antibiotic-associated pseudomembranous colitis.
Indications (Ocular Disease)	Infectious cavernous sinus thrombosis (i.v.), open globe (topical + i.v.), endophthalmitis (all routes of administration), keratitis.
Subconjunctival	25 mg/0.5 ml.
Intravitreal	1 mg/0.1 ml.
Intravenous/Oral	1 g i.v., q12h.

Antifungals

Name   Amphotericin B.
Spectrum   *Aspergillus, Blastomyces, Candida, Coccidioides, Cryptococcus, Histoplasma, Leishmania, Paracoccidioides.*
Indications   Aspergillus canaliculitis, Mucormycosis, Fungal keratitis,
(Ocular Disease)   Fungal endophthalmitis.
Topical   0.1–0.25% solution q1h.
Subconjunctival   0.8–1.0 mg.
Intravitreal   0.005 mg/0.1 ml (5 μg).
Intravenous/Oral   0.25–1.0 mg/kg qd divided into four doses.

Name   Fluconazole.
Spectrum   *Aspergillus, Blastomyces, Candida, Coccidioides, Cryptococcus, Histoplasma.*
Indications   Candida endophthalmitis, Candida albicans canaliculitis.
(Ocular Disease)
Intravenous/Oral   400 mg qd in divided doses for 7–10 days.

Name   Flucytosine.
Spectrum   *Candida, Cryptococcus.*
Indications   Fungal endophthalmitis.
(Ocular Disease)
Topical   1% solution.
Intravenous/Oral   50–150 mg qd divided into four doses.

Name   Itraconazole.
Spectrum   *Acanthamoeba, Aspergillus, Blastomyces, Candida, Coccidioides, Cryptococcus, Histoplasma, Paracoccidioides, Sporothrix, Trichophyton.*
Indications   Aspergillus cancaliculitits, Acanthamoeba keratits, Fungal
(Ocular Disease)   endophthalmitis.
Intravenous/Oral   100–200 mg b.i.d.

Name   Ketoconazole.
Spectrum   *Acanthamoeba, Blastomyces, Candida, Coccidioides, Cryptococcus, Epidermophyton, Histoplasma, Malassezia, Microsporum, Paracoccidioides, Phialophora, Trichophyton.*
Indications   Fungal keratitis, Acanthamoeba keratits.
(Ocular Disease)
Intravenous/Oral   200–400 mg qd.

Name   Natamycin.
Spectrum   *Aspergillus, Candida, Cephalosporium, Fusarium, Penicillium.*
Indications   Fungal keratitis, Fungal blepharoconjunctivitis, Fungal end-
(Ocular Disease)   ophthalmitis.
Topical   5% solution q1h (commercially available).

Name	Voriconazole.
Spectrum	*Aspergillus, Candida, Fusarium, Scedosporium.*
Intravenous/Oral	*IV*: 6 mg/kg q12h for the first 24 h as loading dose, then 4 mg/kg i.v. or 200 mg. *Oral*: q12h as maintenance dose.

Antivirals

Name	Acyclovir sodium.
Spectrum	Herpes simplex virus (HSV), herpes zoster virus (HZV).
Indications (Ocular Disease)	Acute retinal necrosis.
Intravenous/Oral	*IV*: 5–10 mg/k qd divided into three doses until resolution, then 800 mg. *Oral*: five times per day for 1–2 months.
Indications (Ocular Disease)	Progressive outer retinal necrosis syndrome.
Intravenous/Oral	*IV*: 5–10 mg/k qd divided into three doses until resolution, then 800 mg. *Oral*: five times per day for 1–2 months.
Indications (Ocular Disease)	Anterior uveitis (HSV).
Intravenous/Oral	400 mg p.o. five times per day.
Indications (Ocular Disease)	Herpes keratitis.
Intravenous/Oral	400 mg p.o. five times per day for 10 days.
Indications (Ocular Disease)	Prophylaxis of keratitis recurrence.
Intravenous/Oral	400 mg p.o. b.i.d. up to 1 year (longer for corneal graft involvement).
Indications (Ocular Disease)	HSV or HZV eyelid involvement.
Intravenous/Oral	400–800 mg p.o. five times per day for 5–10 days. If immunocompromised, 10–12 mg/kg qd, i.v. in divided into three doses for 10–14 days.
Indications (Ocular Disease)	Herpes zoster choroiditis, optic neuritis, cranial nerve palsy.
Intravenous/Oral	5–10 mg/kg i.v., q8h for 1 week.
Name	Cidofovir.
Spectrum	Cytomegalovirus (CMV).
Indications (Ocular Disease)	CMV retinitis.
Intravenous/Oral	Induction: 5 mg/kg i.v. over 1 hr once weekly for 2 weeks. Maintenance: 5 mg/kg over 1 hr every 2 weeks.
Name	Famciclovir.
Spectrum	HSV, HZV.

Indications **(Ocular Disease)**	HSV or HZO ophthalmicus (HZO) eyelid involvement.
Intravenous/Oral	500 mg t.i.d. for 7 days.
Indications **(Ocular Disease)**	Herpes keratitis (HZO).
Intravenous/Oral	500 mg t.i.d. for 7 days.

Name	Fomivirsen.
Spectrum	CMV.
Indications **(Ocular Disease)**	CMV retinitis.
Intravitreal	165–330 µg every week for 3 weeks then every 2 weeks.
Intravenous/Oral	Induction: 330 µg/0.05 ml i.v. every other week for two doses. Maintenance: 330 µg/0.05 ml i.v. every 4 weeks.

Name	Foscarnet sodium.
Spectrum	CMV, HSV.
Indications **(Ocular Disease)**	CMV retinitis.
Intravitreal	2.4 mg/0.1 ml or 1.2 mg/0.05 ml 2–3 times per week for 2–3 weeks, then 2.4 mg/0.1 ml 1–2 times per week.
Intravenous/Oral	Induction: 90 mg/kg i.v., q12h or 60 mg/kg q8h for 2–3 weeks. Maintenance: 90–120 mg/kg qd.

Name	Ganciclovir sodium.
Spectrum	CMV.
Indications **(Ocular Disease)**	CMV retinitis.
Intravitreal	Pellet implantation: release 1 µg/h (lasts 6–8 months). Intravitreal injection: 200–2,000 µg/0.1 ml two to three injections per week for 2–3 weeks, then 200–2,000 µg/0.1 ml per week.
Intravenous/Oral	Induction: 5 mg/kg i.v., q12h for 14–21 days. Maintenance: 5 mg/kg qd, i.v. 7 days per week, or 6 mg/kg qd 5 days per week, or p.o. 1,000 mg t.i.d., or 500 mg for 6 days (q3h). Concomitant with intravitreal pellet: 1,000–2,000 mg p.o., t.i.d.

Name	Trifluridine.
Spectrum	HSV.
Indications **(Ocular Disease)**	HSV blepharoconjunctivitis or keratitis.
Topical	1% solution every 2 h while awake up to nine times per day until complete epithelialization of corneal ulcer, then every 4 h while awake for a minimum 5 drops qd for 7 days.

Name	Valacyclovir.
Spectrum	HSV, HZV.
Indications **(Ocular Disease)**	Acute retinal necrosis.
Intravenous/Oral	After resolution of retinitis with i.v. acyclovir: 1 g p.o., t.i.d. for 1–2 months.

Indications (Ocular Disease) Intravenous/Oral	Herpes keratitis (HZV).
	1 g p.o., t.i.d. for 7 days.
Indications (Ocular Disease) Intravenous/Oral	HZV eyelid involvement.
	1 g p.o., t.i.d. for 7 days.
Name	Valganciclovir hydrochloride.
Spectrum	CMV.
Indications (Ocular Disease) Intravenous/Oral	CMV retinitis.
	Induction: 900 mg p.o. b.i.d. for 21 days. Maintenance: 900 mg p.o., qd.
Name	Vidarabine (not available in USA).
Spectrum	HSV.
Indications (Ocular Disease) Topical	HSV blepharoconjunctivitis or keratitis.
	3% solution five times per day for 10–14 days.